CHINESE MICRO-MASSAGE

CHINESE MICRO-MASSAGE

Acupuncture Without Needles

by

J. LAVIER

Doctor of Acupuncture (China)
Professor at the Institute of Acupuncture Wu Wei-Ping

THORSONS PUBLISHERS LIMITED
Wellingborough, Northamptonshire

Mi - World
511 W. 49th Street
Hialeah, Fla. 33012

First published in France as *Le Micro-massage Chinois et les techniques qui en dérivent*

© Librairie Maloine S.A., Paris, 1973
First English edition published 1977

ISBN 0 7225 0362 8

Photoset by Specialised Offset Services Ltd., Liverpool
Made and Printed in Great Britain by
Weatherby Woolnough Ltd., Sanders Road,
Wellingborough, Northants.

CONTENTS

PREFACE

One of the oldest medical texts we possess, if not the very oldest, is the *Nei Tching Sou Wen*, the canon of Chinese medicine attributed to Houang Ti (2700 B.C.). The eighty-one chapters of this work, contained in 700 pages of fine ideographic writing, remain even today the sole reference of traditional practitioners in the Far East. In Chapter 12 we read: 'Paralyses and contractures are amenable to massage and gymnastics.'

In modern terms what this concise statement recommends is manual mobilizations (massage) or passive mobilizations (gymnastics) of the muscular groups, according to whether the condition is one of hypertonia (contracture) or hypotonia (paralysis), which is neither more nor less than a precise definition of the techniques of the modern masseur-kinesitherapist.

In China, masso-kinesitherapy was, and is, one of the noble arts of medicine. It is hardly surprising that the ancient Chinese techniques are not very different from those of the modern West, as the anatomical and physiological laws underlying them have been handed down almost unchanged from the China of the third millennium B.C. to our own era, having come to us via Ancient Egypt, Greece and Rome.

However, the Chinese have retained a form of massage which is peculiar to themselves. Technically speaking, it bridges a gap between classical massage and acupuncture. It is termed by us *micro-massage*. The idea of this particular method is the therapeutic exploitation of certain regions of the body – the acupuncture points or dermotopes – by strictly external and physical means. From acupuncture micro-massage borrows the doctrine of peridromes[1] and dermotopes, and from massage its external techniques. Thus the dermotopes are treated by hand or by means of special instruments, but, unlike what happens in acupuncture, without ever breaking the skin.

Westerners have been seriously handicapped in the study of Chinese medicine by lack of direct access to the original texts; so, because acupuncture as practised here is derived from incomplete and often inaccurate translations, it bears little more than a faint resemblance to its Chinese counterpart. And when we come to micro-massage, such descriptions as are available are only fragments of the source works, and even these are travesties rather than translations. It is on such uncertain, feeble and questionable foundations then, that Chinese medicine has been reconstructed in France by authors ignorant of the Chinese language and with no knowledge of the subject with which they are dealing.

This regrettable state of affairs has been in existence since 1930, when there was a birth or revival of unorthodox methods and theories in medical circles. It was then that acupuncture appeared on the scene, shrouded in mystery and supported by sponsors like homoeopathy, chiropractic, osteopathy, radionics and astro-medicine, and was classified under esoteric medicine according to the prevailing fashion. As nobody at that time seemed ever to have set eyes on a true acupuncture needle, the astrologically-minded invented their famous gold and silver pins – instruments 'of the sun and the moon', which had neither been described nor used by Chinese practitioners.

However, the process did not stop with the invention of

---

[1] Usually referred to as the 'meridians', but the author of the present work prefers to adopt the term 'peridrome', as explained in Chapter 2. – *Tr.*

instruments. In default of authentic documentation, new techniques were devised, and acupuncture, having been 're-invented', is now completely distorted and misrepresented, possessing a poetical-cum-mystical basis it has never had in China. So let it be stressed: it is the West which has cheapened Chinese medicine with pseudo-folklorist orientalism.

Our aim should be to keep micro-massage entirely free of such caricature.

Definition of Micro-massage

How can Chinese micro massage best be defined? In the first place it is a form of massage, because it is concerned with the massage of precise regions of the body. But it is miniaturized massage, for these 'regions' are cutaneous zones of very small area, less than a square centimetre – the *dermotopes*, improperly called 'acupuncture points'.

The question arises of how an intervention of this kind, which is mechanically very feeble, can have results equal or even superior to those obtained with classical massage which 'works' the muscle or group of muscles or even the deeper layers of the organism? It is here that we encounter the fundamental difference between the two techniques – classical massage is a *mechanical* action, while micro-massage is an *energizing* action. In the same way that the electrologist stimulates the muscles by applying small electrodes to the 'motor points', the micro-masseur, like the acupuncturist, singles out venter points of the muscles, points of insertion, sensor or motor nerve points, ligamentary points, articular points and organic points.

In China, micro-massage is a technique which has been developed to perfection for a very long time. It is employed not only by specialists but also by the acupuncturists who, confronted by a child or squeamish patient who refuses the needles, will use it to treat the dermotopes indicated. Acupuncturists, in any case, have never thought of micro-massage as being inferior to the method with needles. The only difference is that about three sessions of micro-massage are needed to achieve the same result as is obtained from a single session of acupuncture.

Finally, and in spite of the spectacular results so often obtained by it, Chinese micro-massage is completely harmless apart from a few contra-indications which will be mentioned in the course of this book.

CHAPTER ONE

THE FUNDAMENTAL DUALITY

The usual approach of Western medicine to disease is to concentrate on the disordered organ or function, studying it in isolation as if it enjoyed an independent existence. This way of looking at things has naturally led to the system of specialization: the cardiologist does not explore the digestive tube while the gastro-enterologist is not interested in the cardiovascular functions. Our highly specialized modern practitioners are caught up in analytical abstraction.

It is quite different with the Chinese physician, who travels the pathway of synthesis. An omnipractitioner by definition and by the requirements of theory, he is unable to comprehend the meaning of specialization because, instead of abstracting the diseased organ, he will consider it in its context and examine its regulations with all the other functions. Carrying this method to its logical conclusion, he will then view the organism in its environment and search into the anomalies and relationships there. For, in the words of the Chinese tradition as interpreted by the *Nei Tching Sou Wen*, the organism is closely linked with its environment, being unable to live without it, and only breathes, feeds and excretes with its help. Submerged in the cosmos like a fish in water, it is a compulsory link in the carbon, phosphorus, nitrogen and oxygen cycles, and so on.

Since he depends on it so strongly, man must not only be aware of but must also faithfully reflect the rhythms of his environment in company with all other living things. Hence, he is active during the day and passive during the night, he labours in the fields during the warm season and lies up for the winter, adjusting his behaviour to the most elementary of natural rhythms. This simple observation has suggested to the Chinese that the environmental cycles (those of the macrocosm) are repeated within the organism (the microcosm), which can and must be considered as a miniature universe, resembling the greater universe (in which it is embedded, with which it is integrated, and from which it takes its rhythms) in all points.

The rhythms of the cosmos all seem to form one and the same *pulsation*, susceptible to varying degrees. Thus, the four seasons of the year are perfectly comparable to the four parts of every twenty-four hours:

Year	**24 hours**
Spring	Morning
Summer	Noon
Autumn	Evening
Winter	Night

If we forget for the moment the intermediate 'times' of spring/morning and autumn/evening, it is possible to distinguish a binary rhythm, a regular alternation between noon and night or between summer and winter or, to put it another way, a general rhythm of action and repose obeyed by the organism in common with the whole of nature. That is why, in addition to the great primordial rhythms mentioned above, there is an infinity of submultiple harmonic rhythms, such as the respiratory cycle (inspiration-expiration), the cardiac cycle (systole-diastole), the regular successive states of repletion and depletion of the different organs of the digestive tract, and so on. Finally, the smallest living cell reflects this rhythm in its most elementary metabolism (anabolism-catabolism).

The Yin-Yang System

In order to illustrate this alternating duality, the Chinese have elaborated the *Yin-Yang* system. These terms are extremely general and respectively symbolize action (Yang) and rest or inertia (Yin). Thus, while *Yang* is the essence of summer, day, light, warmth, exteriority, *Yin* is that of winter, night, darkness, cold, interiority. Hence there is a regularly descending scale of *Yin* and *Yang*, from the galactic pulsation, through the succession of the seasons and of night and day, right down to the most rapid vibrations like those of gamma radiations or cosmic rays. This regular alternation is termed *Tao*, the universal law from which the Taoist teaching was derived, the philosophy which prescribes the strictest possible observance of the *Yin-Yang* rhythms for the preservation of good health and the promotion of longevity.

The presence of spring and autumn in the seasonal rhythm and that of morning and evening in the twenty-four hour period, just like the four quarters of a lunation, shows that *Yin* and *Yang* succeed one another not only regularly but progressively as well. They engender one another reciprocally. In order for *Yang* to engender *Yin*, let us say, it needs to contain at least an infinitesimal part of it, from which the Chinese have deduced that there is no such thing as an absolute *Yin* and *Yang*; there is always some *Yang* in the *Yin* and some *Yin* in the *Yang*. Therefore *Yang* really signifies more of *Yang* than *Yin*, and *Yin* implies more of *Yin* than *Yang*.

In the light of this, some idea of the proportions of *Yin-Yang* can be given in the table below:

Year	24 hours	Yin-Yang Proportions
Spring	Morning	50/50
Summer	Noon	1/99
Autumn	Evening	50/50
Winter	Night	99/1

This notion of the *Yin-Yang* 'proportion' is essential if one wants to understand the main principles of Chinese medicine, and in particular those of micro-massage.

Functions of the Organisms

At the date when the *Nei Tching Sou Wen* was compiled – 4,500 years ago according to Chinese chronology – the principal functions of the organism were already known, and were designated by symbols. These symbols are names of organs which Westerners have made the great mistake of taking literally, involving themselves in an inextricable maze of errors in therapeutics. Table 1 on page 16 is the list of these principal functions, of which there are twelve. These will be designated by their initials.

Therefore, as a function is connected with the blood, the internal environment (microcosm) or with the external environment (macrocosm), it is described as *Yin* or as *Yang*.

The *Yang* functions are called *Fou*, e.g. D or E, which are open to the exterior, and the *Yin* functions are called *Tsang*, e.g. C or H, which are not connected with the exterior.

The twelve principal functions are divided into six *Tsang* and six *Fou*, but subgroups can be distinguished inside each of these two groups. In fact, in the *Fou* set, E is certainly more *Yang* than A is, since it is in communication with the exterior; while A does not have this direct contact (ileum and jejunum). In the same way, R is more *Yang* than C, for the same reason.

It will therefore be understood that the Chinese established a *Yin-Yang* hierarchy of the twelve functions in which can be distinguished the peristaltic *Fou* functions and the reservoir *Fou* functions, the periodic *Tsang* functions and the immobile *Tsang* functions. The peristaltic *Fou* functions are animated by continual movements of contraction, whereas the reservoir *Fou* functions have inert periods during which they fill, separated by more or less frequent flushing. Consequently, the peristaltic-*Fou* functions are more *Yang* than the reservoir *Fou* functions.

The *Tsang* functions, on the other hand, are divided into those which are periodic, animated by permanent cyclic movements (R and C), and into immobile *Tsang* functions which have no apparent movements.

Table 2 shows the *Yin-Yang* hierarchy of the functions according to this principle. To make it easy to remember, the approximate *Yin-Yang* ratio is mentioned for each function, showing quite clearly that the *Fou* functions are not strictly speaking *Yang*, but more *Yang* than *Yin*. The same is true, but the other way round, where the *Tsang* is concerned.

It will be noted that P occupies the same place as A in the table, and V, as an annexe of C, is in the same place as C.

Table 1

Organs — symbols	Functions designated	Abbreviations
Fei (lungs)	respiration, lungs, skin	R (respiration)
Ta Tch'ang (colon)	colon, evacuation of faeces	E (evacuation)
Wei (stomach)	salivary glands, oesophagus, stomach, duodenum, pancreas (exocrine)	D (digestion)
Pi (spleen)	leukocytes, erythrocytes, lymphoid organs, lymph, reticulo-endothelial tissue, pancreas (endocrine)	L (lymph)
Sin (heart)	heart and blood pressure	C (heart - cardiac)
Siao Tch'ang (small intestine)	jejunum and ileum, absorption	A (absorption)
P'ang Kouang (bladder)	urinary excretion, urinary passages	U (urinary passages)
Chen (kidney)	adrenals and glomerules, urinary secretion	S.(adrenals - suprarenals)
Sin Pao Lao (vasoconstriction)[1]	vasomotoricity, sympathetic	V (vessels)
San Tcchiao (triple warmer)	the three parts of the parasympathetic system; cardiopulmonary pneumogastric, visceral pneumogastric, pelvic parasympathetic	P (parasympathetic)
Tan (gall bladder)	biliary function of the liver, bile ducts	B (bile)
Kan (liver)	sanguine functions of the liver (iron, glycogen, etc.): hepatic metabolism	H (hepatic functions)

[1] Termed 'circulation — sex' in some English works on acupuncture. *Tr.*

Table 2

Class	Sub-class	Function		Yin-Yan ratio
Fou (*Yang* functions)	peristaltic (*Yang*)	E		1/99
		A	(P)	25/75
	reservoir (*Yin*)	U		30/70
		B		35/65
		D		49/51
	periodic (*Yang*)	R		55/45
		C	(V)	65/35
Tsang (*Yin* functions)	immobile (*Yin*)	L		70/30
		H		75/25
		S		99/1

CHAPTER TWO

THE PERIDROMES

It is not surprising that the Chinese long anticipated us in the discovery of the main physiological functions: this is just what might be expected from the very advanced state of their civilization and knowledge at a time when much of Europe was inhabited by unsophisticated communities. What is astonishing, however, is their conception of the *Tching*, which we are just beginning to discover very tentatively now.

Starting with the principle that the organism is in harmony with its environment, they entered on a painstaking study of the frontier which separates these two worlds – the skin. In fact, the skin possesses an internal microcosmic side and an external macrocosmic side, and must therefore, in the interests of the harmony mentioned, represent each element of the organism so as to put it in contact with the cosmos. Thus arose the idea of *Tching*, the ideogram of which indicates that it is something very thin, running longitudinally, which transports energy. There are twelve pairs of these lines disposed symmetrically on the human body, each pair corresponding to one of the twelve principal functions.

Every active organ, every organ which lives, produces energy, the chemical and electrical manifestations of which are known to us. The originality of the Chinese lay in showing that each function sends a part of its energy to the surface, channelled in its own pair of *Tching*. Thus the *Tching* seems to be a 'track of energy', a kind of invisible conductor, which follows a very precise pathway, for which the translation 'meridian' is not sufficiently exact. We ourselves prefer, with C. Grégory, the term 'drome' (from the Greek *dromos*, a path or way).

The internal pathways by which a function or an organ sends a portion of its energy to the surface have been minutely described by the Chinese and tally with central nervous or vegetative pathways, forming 'nodes' which correspond to the various plexi. So the energy of a function first follows an internal course, or *cryptodrome*, and then traverses the surface of the skin along the *Tching* or *peridrome*, which has the name of the particular function.

The Topography of the Peridromes
It is essential to have a good knowledge of the topography of the peridromes, because these lines pass through the dermotopes treated by acupuncturists and micro-masseurs.[1] In keeping with what would logically be expected from the theory of *Tao*, this topography was soon confirmed by therapeutic experience. In order to understand this properly, we need to return to what was said in the previous chapter and to complete it briefly.

Since *Yang* is that which is external and *Yin* is that which is internal, the back surface will be *Yang* and the front surface *Yin*. Indeed, embryology teaches us that foetal morphology implies an external (*Yang*) dorsal surface and an internal (*Yin*) ventral surface (Figure 1). Consequently, the *Yang* peridromes (relating to the *Fou* functions) will be posterior, while the *Yin* peridromes (relating to *Tsang*) will be anterior.

We are informed by *Taoist* teaching that the heavens, being intangible and in motion, are *Yang*, whereas the earth, being tangible and apparently immobile, is *Yin*. From this it is easy to conclude, with the Chinese, that whatever is above is *Yang* and whatever is below is *Yin*. The upper parts of the body (with the head and thorax, which contain the noble periodic

[1] Diagrams showing the peridromes and dermotopes will be found at the end of the book.

Tsang functions) are more *Yang* than the lower parts (the abdomen and the organs of digestion and excretion) which are more *Yin*.

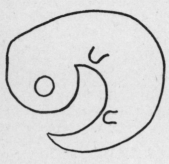

Fig. 1

It is therefore only natural, from the point of view of *Tao*, that the proximal extremities of the peridromes, containing a noble energy, should be found at the top of the body. In addition to this, there are two parts to be distinguished within the top region: the head is more *Yang* (brain, mind) than the thorax (heart, lungs). Consequently, the proximal extremity of all *Yang* peridromes will be at the head, and that of all *Yin* peridromes will be at the thorax.

In locating the distal extremities of the twelve bilateral peridromes, the *Yin-Yang* hierarchy of functions comes into play. The peridromes associated with the most *Yang* of *Tsang* functions and with the most *Yang* of the *Fou* functions have their distal extremity in the hand and concern the upper limb

(*Yang*); the peridromes associated with the most *Yin* of *Tsang* and *Fou* functions have their distal extremity in the foot and concern the lower limb (*Yin*). Therefore, if Table 1 is adapted to the scheme of the peridrome, Table 3 results.

Table 3

Class of function	Proximal extremity of the peridrome	Subclass of the function	Distal extremity of the peridrome	Function	Location of the peridrome
Fou (*Yang*)	face	peristaltic (*Yang*)	hand (upper limb)	E P A	ext. mid. int. } posterior
		reservoir (*Yin*)	foot (lower limb)	U B D	posterior lateral anterior
Tsang (*Yin*)	thorax	periodic (*Yang*)	hand (upper limb)	R V C	ext. mid. int. } anterior
		immobile (*Yin*)	foot (lower limb)	L H S	ext. mid. int. } anterior to the trunk

The nature of the energy of one of the reservoir *Fou* functions, the D function, gives rise to a displacement of the *Yin-Yang* limit at the peridrome level. What is found is that peridrome D is anterior, in spite of its relationship with a *Fou* function. Its proportion of *Yang* relative to *Yin* is so small (see Table 1) that it has a *Yin* topography. Nevertheless, its proximal extremity lies in the head (*Yang*).

The Current of Energy

Each peridrome has a definite direction, which determines which way the current of energy flowing through it will run, and decides the numbering of the dermotopes of which it is composed.

It is possible, then, to distinguish four groups of three peridromes. (Figure 2):

The thorax-hand group comprises peridromes R, C and V.
The hand-head group comprises peridromes E, A and P.
The head-foot group comprises peridromes D, U and B.
The foot-thorax group comprises peridromes L, S and H.

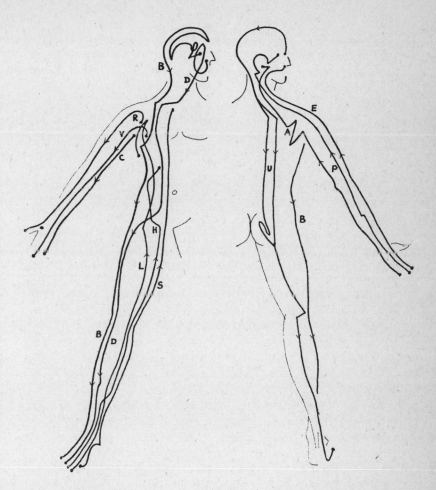

Figure 2
The twelve peridromes on the right side (schematic)

CHAPTER THREE

THE PHYSIOLOGICAL ENERGY SYSTEM OF THE PERIDROMES

The Chinese have only one way of locating the peridromes – by palpation. They are in fact situated along the intermuscular or intertendinous valleys, which are easily traced by the finger. We in the West, who are always looking for evidence, have been unable to discover any anatomical or histological structure capable of justifying these pathways. It is to the electrologists that we owe the desired proof; proof which is not only becoming clear, but indisputable too. They have demonstrated that the ohmic resistance of the skin falls considerably in certain regions for reasons which are still a mystery, and that this modification occurs in every human being. These special regions are those same peridromes, the *Tching* of the Chinese.

What is more, if the course of a peridrome is followed with the help of an exploratory electrode connected to an ohmmeter, it will be found that its resistance, which is already very low, reaches a clear-cut minimum at certain spots. These points of high conductivity are the dermotopes.

Therefore, if the energy of the functions is equated with an electric potential, which is *partly* correct, it will be realized that once this potential has reached the surface it will result in a current and like any other electric current, this will seek out the places of least resistance in which to flow, i.e. the peridromes.

After it had been established by the Chinese that the energy circulated in the peridromes, it was obvious that there had to

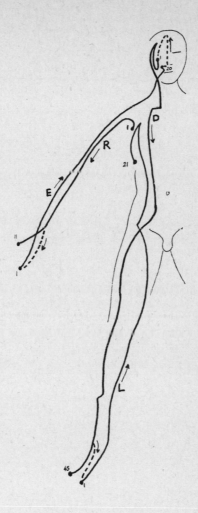

Figure 3
The right REDL circuit
(schematic)

be a high potential in one place and a low potential in another. This circulation is pictured as a variation of the *Yin-Yang* ratio in the energy of the peridromes, and Chinese tradition has proliferated highly refined indications in this regard, of which we shall retain the essentials here.

The energy circulates in the twelve peridromes on one side (it does not matter whether it is the right or the left) following an exact order, in which three circuits each comprising four peridromes can be distinguished. The first circuit is composed of the peridromes R, E, D and L (Figure 3), and the tradition describes it for us as follows:

The energy appears at the first dermotope (thoracic) of the R peridrome and descends to the thumb, to the eleventh and last dermotope of this peridrome. But an anastomosis is derived from the R peridrome at the level of the wrist and proceeds to the first dermotope of the E peridrome, located near the nail of the index finger. By way of this branch, the energy passes into the E peridrome, along which it runs to the twentieth and last dermotope, in the face (next to the nose).

From there, the energy becomes internal, flows to the brain and reappears at the first dermotope of the D peridrome (subocular). Following this centripetal trajectory, the energy will descend to the foot, where the forty-fifth and last dermotope of this peridrome is found, next to the nail of the second toe.

But an anastomosing branch derived from the instep region allows the energy to reach the first dermotope of the L peridrome, near the nail of the big toe, and it makes use of this new pathway to return to the thorax, where, at the level of the twenty-first dermotope of this peridrome (sub-axillary), it disappears 'into the interior'.

The energy will reappear at the surface, after passing through different organs, at the first (thoracic) dermotope of the peridrome which begins the second circuit, and belongs to the same category as the R peridrome, i.e. to the thorax-hand category. It will then flow through this second circuit, in the same way as in the first, in peridromes C, A, U and S, and then through the third, in peridromes V, P, B and H, returning to the first circuit R, E, D, L, etc..

The Head and the Thorax

This peripheral circulation of energy is due to a certain number of factors, the chief of which is a potential difference of energy between the head and the thorax. Figure 4 shows the cycle of the twelve peridromes in three circuits with the numbers allotted to the dermotopes where the energy enters

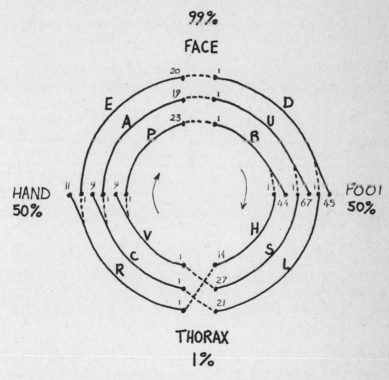

Figure 4
The cycle of the twelve peridromes

and leaves, and also gives the theoretical proportions of *Yang* to *Yin*. The anastomosing branches at the hand and the foot are shown by dotted lines. Dotted lines are also used to show the transfer of the energy to the brain in the face region, and its passage 'to the interior' at the thorax. These dotted lines represent the internal pathways known as cryptodromes.

In reality, the *Yang* maximum is not in the face but in the brain, and its minimum is not in the thorax but 'in the interior of the body'. At thorax level, the afferent peridromes bring in a spent energy (down from 50 per cent to 1 per cent of *Yang*), and the efferent peridromes lead away an energy endowed with a certain growth potential (from 1 per cent to 50 per cent of *Yang*). According to the Chinese, the peripheral energy is 'recharged' by contact with various internal organs, and in particular with the heart, which would accordingly seem to be not only a pump for the blood but an *energy pump* as well.

In passing, it is worth mentioning that Figure 4 confirms the Taoist association of the thorax with winter, of the face with summer, of the hand with spring, and of the foot with autumn. Although the plans differ entirely, the ratio changes are the same.

The Allodromes

Induced by the rhythms of the cosmos and maintained by the cardiac cycle, the variation in energy within the peridromes can present episodic irregularities due either to microcosmic or to macrocosmic events. An over-heavy meal would be an example of a microcosmic perturbation, while a thunderstorm would be a macrocosmic perturbation.

There is a compensating mechanism capable of absorbing these irregularities provided they do not exceed certain limits of tolerance. This mechanism consists of two *Mai* or vessels, unpaired and median, one posterior and the other anterior, each of which is linked to the peridromes by means of cryptodromic anastomoses at different levels. These vessels are median lines of dermotopes identifiable by the usual measurements of the electrical resistance of the skin. Therefore they have a similar structure to that of the peridromes. They differ from these, however, in not being bilateral, and in not being directly integrated with the circuits mentioned above, from which fact they have been given the name *allodromes* (from the Greek *allos*, other, different).

The posterior allodrome is called *Tou*, the governing vessel. Leaving the coccyx to ascend the vertebral column and follow the median line of the head and then the face, it ends in the upper gum. It clearly corresponds to the cerebrospinal axis. Its energy is predominantly *Yang* (posterior localization) and this Governor is none other than the central nervous system. Because of its relationship with an exteriorized function, because of the basically *Yang* energy, and because of the Chinese name Governor or Head (of the family), we shall call it the Male allodrome (M).

The anterior allodrome is called *Jen*, the subordinate, the deputy manager, with the added sense of gestation.[1] This is obviously, in symbolic terms, the female, the wife, in contrast to the Head of the household. Setting out from the perineum, this allodrome ascends the anterior median line of the trunk, and ends at the chin. Its energy is predominantly *Yin* and it corresponds to the autonomic nervous system. This relationship with an interiorized system, its *Yin* energy and its Chinese name implying a contrast with the 'male' allodrome, justifies the nomenclature Female allodrome (F).

The two allodromes, M and F, are joined by a double cryptodrome system which follows the digestive tract and runs to the genital organs. This reinforces them, for it is from this level that they draw their energy, our distinction between male and female.

When there is a lack of energy in the peridromes, the Male (M) allodrome (Governing vessel) supplies the deficiency; conversely, any excess energy is absorbed by the Female (F)

---

[1] Hence the name 'Conception vessel' used in some textbooks. – *Tr.*

allodrome (Conception vessel). However, the compensating action is only effective within certain limits, and if these are exceeded a state of disease exists.

CHAPTER FOUR

ANATROPIC AND CATATROPIC EFFECTS

Strictly speaking, what we have agreed to call the dermotope is only one part of the acupuncture point, the structure of which introduces other concepts; since, although it must be located on the surface as accurately as possible, it must also be located below the surface – at least when needles have to be inserted. This idea of 'sounding' is extremely important in acupuncture, yet it is almost unknown in the West. Each point has a fixed depth, which is a few millimetres for some and several centimetres for others. The whole unit forms a three-dimensional complex called *Hsueh* (hole or well) by the Chinese, and by Westerners (who are only acquainted with the surface location) an acupuncture point, a term from which the notion of depth is absent.

Be that as it may, we know that each peridrome and each allodrome is composed of a precise and invariable number of *Hsueh*, as can be seen in Table 4.

We shall only concern ourselves with the superficial parts of the *Hsueh* (dermotope), since there is no easy access to the deeper parts by the external manipulations of micro-massage.

The energy contained in a peridrome can suffer alterations, whenever perturbations cannot be controlled by the protective system of regulatory and compensating allodromes. These alterations fall into two groups, according to whether they originate in a fault in the energy-emitting function, which then sends a disrupted energy force to its pair of peridromes (microcosmic disturbance), or they originate in some local peripheral symptom (contracture, inflammation, etc. which would be a macrocosmic disturbance), affecting the peridrome directly.

Moreover, these perturbations can be *Yang*, or *Yin*, i.e. they can respond to excesses or to deficiencies of energy. The four pathological cases are summarized in the following table:

Origin of the disorder	*Excess*	*Deficiency*
in the function:	hyperfunction	hypofunction
in the peridrome:	contractures, .	pareses
	inflammations,	atrophies,
	neuralgias, etc.	hypesthesias, etc.

Table 4

Number of *Hsueh* composing
the peridromes on one side
of the body:

R:	11
E:	20
D:	45
L:	21
C:	9
A:	19
U:	67
S:	27
V:	9
P:	23
B:	44
H:	14

Total for one side (right or left):	309
Total for both sides: 309 x 2 =	618
Number of *Hsueh* composing the M allodrome:	28
Number of *Hseuh* composing the F allodrome:	24
Total number of *Hsueh*:	670

The actions performed at the dermotopes are intended to make good the deficiencies or drain the excesses. In Chinese, *Pou* and *Sié* mean 'to reinforce' and 'to drain' respectively, ideas which we shall define more accurately by referring to *anatropic* and *catatropic* effects (from the Greek, *ana*, to augment, and *kata*, to diminish).

When the disorder has a peripheral (peridromic) origin, manipulating the dermotopes of the peridrome will exercise a direct action on the situation. When, on the other hand, the disorder has a central origin at functional level, the action will have an induced effect on the function, the origin of the peridromic energy

Because micro-massage is a technique ancillary to acupuncture, it obeys the same laws, whether of theory or practice.

Special note should be taken of the following rule which, probably owing to an error in translation, has been stated in reverse in some European textbooks: *All anatropic effects result from a quick, light and brief action, and all catatropic effects result from a leisurely, strong and prolonged action.*

At one period, great store was set by rotary massage, the effect of which was believed to be anatropic or catatropic according to the direction of rotation. The question of the reality of the supposed effect applies equally to the effect of rotating an acupuncture needle, and the Chinese are still debating it. In fact, the concept is relatively modern and there is no consensus of opinion as to which is the anatropic and which the catatropic direction. For some authors, the positive (clockwise) sense is anatropic and the negative (anticlockwise) sense is catatropic. For others the reverse is true. In the interests of brevity, I have translated a recent study by my colleague Tsouei Tchieh of Taiwan, which illustrates the differences that exist on this subject in the various classical Chinese treatises. Table 5 is an exact translation of the Table he has given in his work, *Tchen Tchiou Pou Sié Fa Ti Li Loun Yu Cheu Tchi (The Theory and Practice of Anatropic and Catatropic*

Table 5

Person	Time	Side	Peridromes / Effect	I Sue Jou Men Ana	Cata	Tchen Tchiou Ta Tch'eng Ana	Cata	Tchu Ying Ana	Cata	Chen Ying Tching Ana	Cata	Tchen Tchiou Fou Ana	Cata	Chen Tchen Pa Fa Ana	Cata	Hsia Cheou Pa Fa Ana	Cata
MAN	Morning	Left side	hand-head	+	−	+	−										
			thorax-hand	−	+	−	+			−	+						
			head-foot	−	+	+	−										
			foot-thorax	+	−	−	+										
		Right side	hand-head	−	+	+	−										
			thorax-hand	+	−	−	+	+	−	+	−						
			head-foot	+	−	+	−										
			foot-thorax	−	+	−	+										
			Allodrome F							−	+						
			Allodrome M							+	−	+	−				
	Afternoon	Left side	hand-head	−	+	+	−										
			thorax-hand	+	−	−	+			−	+						
			head-foot	+	−	+	−										
			foot-thorax	−	+	−	+										
		Right side	hand-head	+	−	+	−										
			thorax-hand	−	+	−	+	+	−	+	−						
			head-foot	−	+	+	−										
			foot-thorax	+	−	−	+										
			Allodrome F							−	+						
			Allodrome M							+	−			−	+	+	−
WOMAN	Morning	Left side	hand-head	−	+	+	−										
			thorax-hand	+	−	−	+			−	+						
			head-foot	+	−	+	−										
			foot-thorax	−	+	−	+										
		Right side	hand-head	+	−	+	−										
			thorax-hand	−	+	−	+	+	−	+	−						
			head-foot	−	+	+	−										
			foot-thorax	+	−	−	+										
			Allodrome F							+	−						
			Allodrome M							−	+	+					
	Afternoon	Left side	hand-head	+	−	+	−										
			thorax-hand	−	+	−	+			−	+						
			head-foot	−	+	+	−										
			foot-thorax	+	−	−	+										
		Right side	hand-head	−	+	+	−										
			thorax-hand	+	−	−	+	+	−	+	−						
			head-foot	+	−	+	−										
			foot-thorax	−	+	−	+										
			Allodrome F							+	−						
			Allodrome M							−	+						

Effects in Acupuncture). It needs no comment.

The truth about these rotations, which, as has already been said, are anyway of recent origin (going back no further than a few hundred years), lies buried at present beneath this mass of contradictions. We ourselves are unable to discover it. But let us turn now to one well-established, traditional fact accepted by all the authors, both ancient and modern, which is that starting from a dermotope, the massage should follow the peridrome and end one or two centimetres away from the said dermotope. It will at least be clear that one ought to know whether the massage has to be centripetal or centrifugal, whether it has to retreat from or approach the extremities. This matter will be dealt with in the following chapter.

Massage with the Finger Tip

To Westerners the hand is the obvious instrument of massage, but for the Chinese it is axiomatic that micro-massage is performed with the finger tip. As a matter of fact, the finger tip is where the energy is almost in equilibrium and the proportions of *Yin* and *Yang* nearly equal – producing a kind of energic neutrality at the end of the finger, a condition which is peculiarly adapted for the absorption of excess energy or the provision of energy when there is a deficiency.[1] For practical reasons, the pad of the thumb is used, the other digits being less convenient. I have heard that some Western practitioners attribute a special influence to each of the fingers. The Chinese have never alluded to any such influence as far as I know, and I think the idea originates from certain doctrines of astrology and animal magnetism which are not Chinese at all, as is also the case with those gold and silver acupuncture needles already mentioned.

Since the toes are also the seat of an equilibrium of energy, it might be thought that certain foot massage techniques have been derived from Chinese methods. There is no truth in this,

[1] See Chapter 3 and Figure 4.

however, because micro-massage is too precise to be carried out with the toes. Why some lady practitioners in the Far East use their feet to stimulate the erotogenic dermotopes of their clients is for the simple reason that in China the female foot is the most secret part of the body, which is never displayed, and has therefore become a sex object. All this has nothing to do with medical micro-massage!

CHAPTER FIVE

THE GENERAL TECHNIQUE OF MICRO-MASSAGE

Having discarded rotary massage, which is of doubtful origin, and of contradictory techniques, we shall confine ourselves to that which is tested and true: *action along the peridrome, applied from the point of the dermotope outwards and ceasing a few centimetres distant from it*. However, the question is to know whether the massage should be centripetal or centrifugal, and this point is one of extreme importance, since *the direction of the massage determines whether the effect is anatropic or catatropic*.

In order to understand the underlying principle, we shall have to look at the energetics of peridrome physiology.

In the peridromes of the thorax-hand group (R, C, V), the proportion of *Yang* to *Yin* varies from 1 per cent (in the thorax) to 50 per cent (in the hand). Since our action must follow the natural tendency of the variation in energy, anatropic massage will be centrifugal here (towards the hand), in the direction of an increasing *Yang* ratio, while catatropic massage will be centripetal (towards the shoulder), in the direction of a decreasing *Yang* ratio.

In the peridromes of the hand-head group (E, A, P), the proportion of *Yang* to *Yin* varies from 50 per cent (in the hand) to 99 per cent (in the head). The anatropic massage will therefore be centripetal here (towards the face), in the direction of an increasing *Yang* ratio, and the catatropic massage will be centrifugal (towards the hand), in the direction of a decreasing *Yang* ratio.

In the peridromes of the head-foot group (D, U, B), the

proportion of *Yang* to *Yin* decreases from 99 per cent (in the head) to 50 per cent (in the feet). Hence, here the anatropic massage will be centripetal (towards the face), in the direction of an increasing *Yang* ratio, and the catatropic massage will be centrifugal (towards the feet), in the direction of a decreasing *Yang* ratio.

In the peridromes of the foot-thorax group (L, S, H), the proportion of *Yang* to *Yin* decreases from 50 per cent (in the foot) to 1 per cent (in the thorax). Thus the anatropic massage will be centrifugal here (towards the foot), in the direction of an increasing *Yang* ratio, and the catatropic massage will be centripetal (towards the thorax), in the direction of a decreasing Yang ratio.

These data are summarized in Figure 5.[1]

Determining the Direction of Passage

The rule which specifies the direction of the massage of a dermotope is called *Yin-Souei* in Chinese – up-stream or down-stream.

The pad of the right thumb is pressed into the peridrome at the dermotope, moves in the direction indicated and is released after traversing one or two centimetres. At that moment, the left thumb is placed on the dermotope (the point of departure) and acts in its turn, to be followed by the right thumb again, and so on. Thus the dermotope experiences a continuous action imparted by the alternate operation of the two thumbs.

It will bear frequent repetition, so it can be repeated here, that an anatropic effect results from rapid, light massage (effleurage), while forceful, deep, slow massage produces a catatropic effect.

[1] Although there is seldom any application for the following, it should be noted that for the allodrome F the catatropic direction is centrifugal and the anatropic direction is centripetal, while for the allodrome M the catatropic direction is centripetal and the anatropic direction is centrifugal (direction defined in relation to the head).

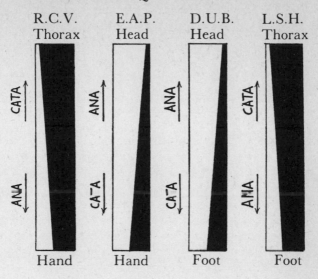

Figure 5
The directions of micro-massage
(Yang in white and Yin in black)

Perhaps the idea will be more easily conveyed by the statement that the aim of anatropic massage is to give warmth to a dermotope lacking in energy, while strong, slow pressure (which must not heat the skin) is used to drain excess energy, expelling it from the point of pressure in the direction of the decreasing proportion of *Yang*.

Instruments
The above may be regarded as the original technique of Chinese micro-massage, a technique which has since been slightly modified, especially in the last hundred years or so. Experience has shown that results are improved if, instead of

using the pad of the finger, the flat of the nail is employed (preferably the nail of the bent index finger). The horny material of the nail is an electric insulator or dielectric; and it is interesting to note that this very special tissue is found only at the extremities of the fingers and toes, where there is no manifestation of peridrome energy, the latter being in a state of equilibrium with equal proportions of *Yang* (activity) and *Yin* (inertia).

The genuine Chinese acupuncture needle is not that little pin of precious metal which is being imposed on the West, but a bimetallic instrument formed of a shaft of steel (iron) and a handle of copper. The essential bimetallism produces a thermo-electric couple which, according to the state of the *Hsueh* on which it acts, endows electrons (negative electricity) when there is excess energy (a positive electrical state) or, on the other hand, removes electrons when energy is deficient (a negative electrical state). But, in accordance with the principle exemplified by the amber rod when rubbed by a cloth or on the skin (it is from the Greek name for amber, *elektron*, that our word electricity is derived) – a principle on which numerous electrostatic machines are based – an insulator (dielectric) under the action of friction, donates electrons to or takes them away from the material with which it is rubbed.

A principle such as this would explain to a great extent the effects of Chinese micro-massage, given the electrical characteristics of the peridromes and dermotopes, the latter in fact being points of concentration of the peridromic potential.[2]

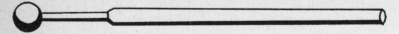

Figure 6
Yuan Tchen

[2] This is why the Chinese micro-masseur never works on skin covered in grease – he needs it to be dry. Talc can be used, but grease, being an electrical insulator, is strongly discouraged.

Consequently, friction with a special instrument will be preferred to manual massage even when done with the nail. The instrument in question was initially a little ivory ball, which was later fitted with a handle to facilitate its manipulation. It is called *Yuan Tchen* – the blunt-tipped instrument (Figure 6).

The *Yuan Tchen* is especially adapted for cataropic treatments (slow and deep). It is equally possible to use it for light and rapid effleurages in anatropic treatments, but other methods and instruments are preferred to reinforce deficient energy in the dermotopes.

CHAPTER SIX

THE FORMS OF CUTANEOUS STIMULATION

Yang is active and *Yin* is passive. To illustrate this definition, suppose we pick up a book and hold it in front of us at arm's length. The book does not move. It has constant mass, which is being acted on both by gravity and by the force we apply to it in counteracting its weight. In other words, *Yang* (the applied force) equalizes Yin (weight).

If we lift the book, the applied force now becomes stronger than the weight, which remains unchanged – and the *Yang* is superior to the *Yin*. If, on the other hand, the book is lowered, the applied force becomes less than the weight – and the *Yang* is inferior to the *Yin* which remains unchanged throughout.

This simple example, although very straightforward, will help us to understand that on the plane or peridromic energy it is always possible for us to act on the *Yang* (the force) but never on the *Yin* (the weight, or rather the mass, the intrinsic, non-modifiable quality). All the interventions of acupuncture, of micro-massage and of their derivative techniques, *are aimed at modifying the Yin-Yang ratio by acting solely on the Yang*, which is the only accessible and modifiable element of the fundamental binary.

When we speak of an excess of energy, or *Yang* condition, we mean an abnormally high proportion of *Yang* in respect of *Yin*; and deficiency, or the *Yin* condition, is no more than a very low proportion of *Yang* in respect of *Yin*. This enables us to define the two great states *Cheu* and *Hsu*, excess and deficiency, and their various modalities, with more precision (Figure 7).

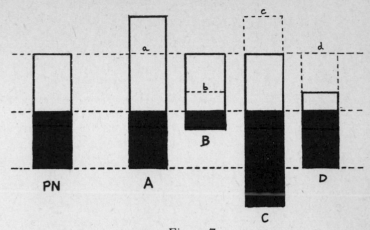

Figure 7

Pathological modifications of the Yin-Yang ratio (Yang in
white and Yin in black)

We shall assume a normal *Yang-Yin* ratio as a standard of
reference. In the diagram, this normal proportion (PN) will be
50 per cent for the sake of simplicity. However, it could just as
well have had some other value, since the proportion varies
according to the peridrome and dermotope in question.

A *Cheu* condition, or excess of energy, signifies too much
Yang in relation to *Yin*. A case like this can present two very
different aspects: either excess *Yang* with normal *Yin* (A), or
normal *Yang* with deficient *Yin* (B). Since, by definition, we
cannot act on the *Yin*, all we can do in either case is to restore
the *Yang* (by catatropic action) to level *a* in case A, and to level
b in case B. The normal proportion will accordingly be
restored but there is no question here of altering the *Yang*
quantitatively, merely its proportion in relation to the *Yin* (50
per cent in our example).

A *Hsu* condition, or deficiency of energy, signifies
inadequate *Yang* in relation to *Yin*. Here again, there are two
possible cases: either normal *Yang* with excess *Yin* (C), or
deficient *Yang* with normal *Yin* (D). Hence it will be necessary

(as we are unable to act on the *Yin*) to restore the *Yang* level – which is the object of anatropic treatment. But it will be observed that whereas in case D it is sufficient to bring the *Yang* back to level *d* when normalizing the proportion of *Yin* to *Yang*, in case C it is necessary to lift it beyond the normal level until it has reached level *c*. While there is only one catatropic method, the sole object of which is to suppress part of the *Yang*, there are two anatropic methods, one for restoring the normal *Yang* level (case D) and the other for producing a *supplement of Yang* so that the latter will rise above its normal level (case C).

The Subcutaneous Puncture

Apart from acupuncture, slow and deep catatropic micro-massage is the only surface body treatment capable of draining excess energy (too much *Yang* in relation to *Yin*) in any given case (either A or B).

On the other hand, anatropic micro-massage (a light and rapid effleurage) can very often restore the *Yang* to its normal level (case D), although it can never boost it beyond this level (case C). In the first case, another method is now preferred which gives quicker and more reliable results. The method is called *P'i Fou Tchen* or subcutaneous puncture.

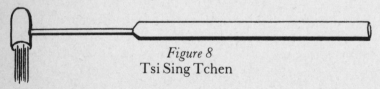

Figure 8
Tsi Sing Tchen

What happens is that the dermotope is stimulated by means of rapid prodding with the point of a lance-shaped needle (*Ts'ai Tchen*). This needle does not break the skin, and the effect is obtained by rubefaction.

In order to bring about this rubefaction more quickly (all anatropic actions have to be of short duration), the Chinese have increased the number of needles and have created a kind of little hammer with a head of seven points, called either the *Tsi Sing Tchen* or seven-point instrument, or the *Ts'oung Tchen* or bunch of needles (Figure 8). Rapid tapotement on the dermotope with this instrument produces rubefaction very quickly, which is a sign of the return of a normal proportion of *Yang*.[1]

However, when it is desired to induce the *Yang* to exceed its normal value in order to balance a *Yin* which is too large (case C), it is obviously necessary to introduce a supplementary energy. This is the aim of the *Tchiou* method, slow cautery.

A distinction must be drawn here between the techniques of *Tchouang* and *Ai Tchuan*, which respectively mean burning or heating at a distance. The burning treatment (*Tchouang*) is carried out on the dermotope with a little cone of dried and powdered artemisia leaves which burn slowly after lighting (moxibustion). This method comes under acupuncture rather than micro-massage, and will not be discussed here because it requires the observance of certain precautions.

On the other hand, heating at a distance is painless and carries no risk of burns with it. As it leaves no mark, it will be the method of choice when one has to deal with a case in which the *Yang* has to be brought above its normal value, an effect which is easily produced by the application of warmth.

The procedure is to heat the dermotope by means of a cigarette of artemisia (*Ai Tchuan*). Thoroughly dried artemisia leaves are pounded in a mortar until a very compact and very fine mass is obtained from which all stalks are carefully removed. This is then ready for rolling into a cigarette. Some Chinese authors recommend that other plants be added to the artemisia in varying proportions, and there are numerous formulas, recently recorded by my colleague Tchwang Yeou-Ming in his new book on acupuncture.

In China such cigarettes are marketed ready-made as

---

[1] Do not forget to sterilize the instrument and the patient's skin with alcohol before treatment.

patent brands, but the essential ingredient of all these formulas is the plant artemisia. My friend Wu Wei-P'ing has tested a large number of combustible materials on the dermotopes and has shown that, all things being equal, it is artemisia which remains the material of choice. As far as I can see, there is no need to attribute some innate occult power to this plant in this particular application. I am inclined to think, after carrying out some laboratory tests, that it is the combustible which, on becoming incandescent, emits the most effective range of infra-red radiation for the desired result, i.e. it gives off an abundance of short wavelengths.

Thus, when the glowing end of the artemisia cigarette is brought close to the dermotope and held at a reasonable distance for 'comfortable warmth' for a certain time, all that is being done is to give a very localized and concentrated application of infra-red rays of excellent quality. Here again, the effect is obtained from the rubefaction of the dermotope.

Diagnosis for Micro-massage

The diagnosis of cases of excess raises no problems. All contractures, all spasms, all pain and all 'hyper' symptoms will be *Yang*, and therefore amenable to catatropic micro-massage. On the other hand, although the signs of deficiency, all 'hypo' conditions (pareses, paralyses, etc.) are *Yin* symptoms, it is still necessary to decide the category of the insufficiency, C or D as in Figure 7, for the method to be employed depends on this decision.

Paralysis, to take one example, is in a state of *Yin*. But as we can only act on the *Yang*, we need to enquire into the condition of the latter. Lax paralysis has very little *Yang* and is included in case D. The appropriate treatment for it is with pricking instruments. But spastic paralysis does show some *Yang* as evidenced by the contracture. Therefore it comes under case C and calls for heat treatment, preferably. The reader who understands this general rule will be able to apply it to all the *Yin* cases which he will meet in everyday practice.

CHAPTER SEVEN

HOW TO USE THE LOCAL DERMOTOPES

Now that the general principles of the micro-massage technique and the methods which complete it are understood, we are in a position to study the very precise laws governing the prescription of the dermotopes. In acupuncture, there are ten rules of prescription (*Cheu Fa*) indicating the dermotopes to treat in any individual case. We shall confine our attention to some only, for we are not concerned with those relating to organic treatment.

The simplest case is that of pricking pain. This could be any sharp pain, *provided it is sited in a dermotope*. Admittedly, some Western authors advise first-aid treatment of any painful point even if it is not a dermotope, but the Chinese frown on all puncture or massage of any point (called by them *T'ien Ying*) which is not a dermotope. When a dermotope is painful, whether spontaneously or under pressure, it is unwise to massage it catatropically right away. Gradual finger pressure should be applied for a minute or two initially, to see if this simple manipulation relieves the pain to any extent. If a start is made on catatropic massage proper at this stage, it will be less uncomfortable than if it had been undertaken immediately.

Pain Away from a Dermotope
If a sharp pain occurs at a *T'ien Ying* point (i.e. at a point which is not a dermotope), the pain itself should not be treated; neighbouring dermotopes should be selected and

treated so as to surround and isolate this painful point. Say a sharp pain occurs in the postero-external side of the arm, in the vastus externus muscle, halfway between the neck and the posterior fold of the armpit: the nearest surrounding dermotopes (P. 12, E. 13 or E. 14) will be chosen and given immediate treatment – in this case, catatropically (centrifugally here).

Apart from this precise case, the rule of the *circle of dermotopes* will be applied in treating areas which do not consist of dermotopes and also in treating zones where the skin and the underlying tissues are in an abnormal condition. In fact, the treatment of dermotopes situated in inflamed or swollen areas or on epidermic lesions is always contra-indicated. What is more, since the dermotopes no longer exist where there are scars, this rule also holds good for scarred regions.

Treating a whole Segment of Peridrome

Sometimes a longitudinal symptom affects a whole segment of peridrome. Although there will be the temptation to massage it all the way along, it is necessary to treat each dermotope in such a segment separately. Sciatica will require catatropic action on each dermotope in the series U.25 to U.30 then as far as U.54 and, if necessary, on the succeeding dermotopes from U.55 to U.60. Anterior tibial paralysis is treated by using the series D.36 to D.39.

It will be recalled that not only must each dermotope be treated separately but the order of their successive treatment will depend on whether the intervention is centripetal or centrifugal. There is a single exception to this rule for treating *dermotopes in series*, and that is cubital neuralgia of the wrist. Because dermotopes C.4, 5, 6 and 7 are so close to one another, the whole series is treated in a single movement (centripetal in this case).

'Dermotopes in Opposition' Rule

Certain loco-regional symptoms call for the application of the *dermotopes in opposition* rule. The procedure here is to choose two opposed dermotopes, generally in a limb segment, one being anterior and the other posterior, or one facing away from and the other facing towards the body. It is essential for the two dermotopes chosen to be situated at exactly the same level, *at the same height*. Usually, this pair of opposed dermotopes will be treated by contrary actions. On the arm, an anatropic manipulation of R.4, an anterior dermotope, and a catatropic manipulation of P.12, a posterior dermotope (these two dermotopes being situated at the same level in relation to the flexural fold of the elbow) stimulate the flexors and relax the extensors of the forearm.

Here we encounter an extremely important mode of treatment because, whenever we act upon any given muscular group, we have to employ a balancing inverse action on the antagonist group.

Vertebral Series of Dermotopes

The plates at the end of this book show the regular and metameric arrangement of the paramesial dorsal dermotopes belonging to peridrome U and at this point the series nearest the vertebral column, running from U.11 to U.26, should be noted. Apart from their action on the internal organs, due to their connection with the ganglions of the sympathetic chain, these dermotopes have a local action on the dorsal muscles.

Considering the obvious fact that the static equilibrium of each vertebra is the result of different forces, chiefly muscular ones, it is easy to understand that what is conventionally called a 'blockade' results from a disturbance of this equilibrium of forces: in short, there is a contraction on one side and a relaxation on the other.

Consequently, an action on the two *symmetrical dermotopes* found on either side of the affected vertebra can restore this vertebra to its normal position in certain very precise conditions of operation. These conditions are quite clear. It is necessary to exercise, in this order, a catatropic action on the side of the contraction and an anatropic action on the relaxed side. This is another application of the principle of antagonistic effects mentioned earlier. As far as the rule of the symmetrical use of dermotopes is concerned, we shall find a further application for it in the next chapter.

CHAPTER EIGHT

SPECIAL DERMOTOPIC INDICATIONS

The previous chapter dealt with local intervention only. This is necessary of course, but sometimes it has to be reinforced by action at a distance, or even replaced by such action. Appreciation of the importance of this point will be helped by the following example.

Pain in the right lumbar region, for which the exact dermotope is U.23, first requires pressure on this dermotope and then catatropic massage of it (centrifugal in this case). This treatment will alleviate the pain and even suppress it, but the latter is always liable to return fairly soon if the excess has not been driven out sufficiently far to be absorbed by the regulatory allodromes. In order to ensure that it goes where it can be taken up by certain energizing anastomoses, preparatory action is necessary before the main treatment, the aim being to attract the energy so as to create a potential difference at a certain distance capable of absorbing the excess expelled by the catatropic massage.

This is why we start the treatment with an anatropic action on dermotope U.54, situated in the popliteal hollow on the right side (the side of the peridrome affected). A series of pricks to the point of rubefaction will accumulate the energy of the peridrome in this dermotope, creating an energy gap above it which will attract the energy forced out of U.23.

Conversely, certain anatropic actions which induce the energy to accumulate in the dermotope treated will be prepared by prior catatropic action at a distance on the same peridrome, the aim of which is to drive the energy towards the dermotope which is in a state of insufficiency.

This rule has very precise conditions of application.

Since the action at a distance must be applied first, before the main local action, the rule regarding the direction of the massage (Chapter 5, Figure 5) enables us to state that it is only possible on the hand-head peridromes (E,A,P) and head-foot peridromes (D,U,B) for a *local* catatropic effect, and on the thorax-hand (R,C,V) peridromes and foot-thorax peridromes (L,S,H) for a *local* anatropic effect.

In addition, the choice of the remote dermotope is governed by the following law:

When the local dermotope is situated towards the proximal extremity of the peridrome (head or thorax), act at a distance on the dermotope which is most distal to this peridrome (finger or toe). Frontal sinusitis, for instance, requires a local catatropic action on U.2 on the upper margin of the orbit, with a preparatory action at a distance (anatropic) on U.67 on the fifth toe.

When the local dermotope is not situated towards the proximal extremity of the peridrome, act at a distance on the dermotope in this peridrome which is located nearest the elbow or knee. An attack of neuritis requiring catatropic action on P.15 (shoulder) will need preliminary treatment of an anatropic nature on P.10 (elbow).

Local or Remote Dermotopes?

The Chinese practitioners are so wedded to this principle of *remote dermotopes* that they think it elegant to avoid overdirect, local treatment. In this they remind one of certain billiard players who feel they have let themselves down if their ball does not touch three cushions before cannoning the two others.

In all cases where a catatropic effect is required, excess energy is more easily drained towards the extremities, which is why, in fact, the remote dermotopes, whether by themselves or in association with the local dermotopes, are rarely employed in peridromes where the catatropic direction is centripetal. This is to avoid releasing the *Yang* in the opposite direction, which is something to be attempted only by practitioners who are very experienced in micro-massage and acupuncture technique.

Paralysis

A final, and very special, indication is that of symmetrical dermotopes treated alternately in the case of unilateral paralysis. All paralysis is characterized by a considerable lack (or even absence) of energy in the peridromes concerned – here on the paralytic side. Logical as it may appear to apply anatropic action to the local dermotopes on the side affected, the energy imparted is nevertheless not enough, and the Chinese advocate similar anatropic action on the corresponding dermotopes *on the sound side of the body*. When the healthy peridrome branch is treated it will become saturated with energy and the body's own energy reserves can be directed to the deficient branch in full concentration. So the micromasseur, like the acupuncturist, treats unilateral paralysis now on the diseased side and now on the healthy side, in an alternating rhythm. The reasons for this will be readily understood from what has just been said.

In cases of paralysis and paresis, heat treatment as described in Chapter 6 will be used on dermotope M.12 in addition to massage and re-education, especially in all medullary and cerebral attacks.

CHAPTER NINE

CHINESE RHEUMATOLOGY

Since this book is intended first and foremost for masseurs and kinesitherapists, it would be impossible to exclude the subject of rheumatism from its pages. A vast amount of ink has been consumed in the West by those writing on this question, and the definition of rheumatism has been debated endlessly. For my own part, I shall refrain from contributing any personal opinions to the controversy but shall confine myself to sketching in broad outline the syndrome termed by the Chinese *Fong Cheu Han Ping*, or, by a euphonic contraction, *Fong Cheu Ping* – the disease caused by wind, cold and damp. Under this clinical heading, a repertory has been compiled of a great number of disorders having in common the fact that they are due to physical agents.

Several years ago, Wu Wei-P'ing devoted a small volume to the *Fong Cheu Ping* syndrome and this has been drawn heavily upon for the bulk of what is said in this chapter and the next.

Energy Imbalance
From the first appearance of the sciences and arts of medicine in China, the wind (*Fong*), the cold (*Han*) and the damp (*Cheu*), which are three natural external enemies of the organism, have been recognized as the three main causes of rheumatism. However, it was realized at the same time that these external factors are incapable of initiating the disease (*Ping*) by themselves. Although they are essentially aggressive, the organism may or may not capitulate in the face of their

attack and invasion. From this has arisen the notion of an internal predisposing cause, an energy imbalance which renders the organism receptive to these external agents. Only the conjunction of the two factors, the one macrocosmic and the other microcosmic, can bring about the *Fong Cheu Ping* syndrome.

One of the ways in which the energy of the peridromes manifests itself is in forming a defence against various external agents. This sentinel role (*Wei*), on which Carrel laid such stress, is seen as vasomotor and thermic phenomena and also as perspiration. Some time during the Song dynasty, Yen Yung-Yao expressed the view that 'the *Fong Cheu Ping* is due to a deficiency in the energy of the skin, the weakened functions (*Ts'ou Li*) of which permit agents such as wind, coldness and humidity to invade the organism'.

In the Ming dynasty, Tchang Yang-San gave the reasons for this reduction in energy when he said: 'The man himself is weakened internally owing to a lack of biological discipline. The external assailants no longer have any difficulty in permeating the organism, and numerous disorders, in particular aches and pains, result from this permeation.'

Wu Wei-P'ing has discerned what is the internal predisposing cause in the tired, the debilitated, the melancholy and in those who over-indulge in alcholic drinks. 'A disorganization of the organism's energy system,' he says, 'paves the main way for attacks on the tissues and joints.'

The external causes which can act as triggers are many and various. The author mentions sudden changes in the weather, clothing which is unsuitable for the climate and season, incidental exposure to wind or rain, the habitat of humid regions, etc. Whether the culprit is water vapour (vapour baths), the exposure of an overheated body to cold, or nothing more than a current of air during sleep (while the energy is quiescent), there is always some abnormal external energy, unexpected in the usual context, which takes advantage of the slightest opportunity to invade the organism by over-running its reduced defences. The sequel is swellings, pain, stiffness and spasms.

The Symptoms of Rheumatism

Yen Yong-Ho (in the Song dynasty) has left us a very poetic description of the first signs of rheumatism: 'The bones,' he said, 'always seem to be too heavy and the limbs are hard to move. The blood flows but poorly, behaving as if it were frozen in the vessels. The joints lose their full play and the muscles experience stiffness.'

Lou Ying's medical treatise describes the wandering pains of the initial attack thus: 'the pain can do nothing more than traverse a region. It moves through it without settling there and goes on to another and so on.'

For Tchang Tching-Yao (in the Ming dynasty), it is the energy of the wind which is responsible for the functional difficulty; that of the cold is responsible for pain by slowing the circulation, and that of humidity is responsible for infiltrations. And Cheng Tchi-Tsong states: 'if the *Yang* dominates in the three aggressive energies, the symptoms will be variable, fugitive and erratic. But if the *Yin* dominates the signs will be those of fixity, stasis and obstruction.' In the work written by Cheou Yao Kang Jou rheumatic symptoms which are *Yang* in character are all listed under the term *Fong*, and all the rheumatic symptoms which are *Yin* in character are given under the term *Pi*.

Fong Cheu Ping can present two distinct clinical aspects, the one chronic, the other acute. If the aspect is chronic, the patient's face looks tired, his muscles are stiff and he finds movement painful and difficult. Aggravations of the symptoms often occur at some fixed hour of the day or night or after any kind of exercise, and also under the influence of wind, cold or damp. In a case such as this inflammatory-type phases are the exception.

In acute cases, the start of the disease is always marked by pain; either by lightning pains right away or by more progressive pain. The parts affected present signs of inflammation, swelling and local heat.

Chinese tradition describes five cardinal groups of symptoms in *Fong Cheu Ping*:

Pain:
This pain (*Souan-T'ong*) can vary a lot. It can be boring, stinging, burning, tearing. Where the superficial tissues are affected, it accompanies swelling.

Disordered sensibility:
The disorders here are of two sorts: either the patient has sensations of formication or of electric tingling, and this is the *Ma* symptom; or else he suffers from hypoaesthesia or even anaesthesia, and this is the *Mou* symptom.

Swelling:
A distinction is made between *Tchong*, or superficial swelling, which only involves the skin and the underlying cellular tissue, and *Tchang*, involving the muscular levels.

Spasms:
The spasm called *Tching* is restricted to the muscular regions bordering the insertions, and leads to a certain limitation of movement; the spasm known as *Tch'iang* involves a whole limb, which, rigid and hard, is rendered powerless.

Paresis and atrophy:
In paresis (*Wei*), the limb is soft and virtually useless. This is the form of the symptom which is most amenable to treatment. Atrophy arises from an old chronic process, the result of a true paralysis. Chinese clinical medicine describes 'the hen's claw' and 'the crane's leg' conditions.

Finally, there exists one last picture, and a particularly grim one, called *T'an-T'ouan*, in which all the tissues are affected – the skin, muscles, tendons, bones, either in a limb or over the entire body. The penetration is general, reaching such organs as the heart, the lungs, the liver, the uterus, etc. It is, says Wu Wei P'ing, the most serious form, and is the likely outcome of a neglected rheumatism.

CHAPTER TEN

THE TREATMENT OF RHEUMATISM

The previous chapters showed the way in which the Chinese approach those very frequent cases of arthritis, arthrosis, neuritis, etc. which are rheumatic in origin. In such cases, acupuncturists employ a special method called *Wen Tchen*, the heated needle. In this, the needle remains in place for at least twenty minutes after insertion and its stem is heated every five minutes by a process we are not now concerned with. Thus the dermotope is subjected to a double effect: a catatropic effect from the duration of implantation and an anatropic effect from the heating. The catatropic effect is directed against the abnormal external energy lodged in the peridrome, drains it (*Sié* and prevents its diffusion to the corresponding function, while the anatropic effect is aimed at reinforcing (*Pou*) the deficient peridromic energy, and thus at restoring its defensive function. We shall do the same in micro-massage.

There are certain specific dermotopes which act selectively on rheumatic disorders. It is useful to have a good knowledge of them, for they will be employed much more often than the others. Because they are so specialized, there is no need to sustain them by action at a distance, and this makes the technique for rheumatism that much simpler. The formulas quoted below will be used, and the effectiveness of these needs no further demonstration.

With symptoms resulting from a first attack (wandering pains), begin by treating the organism in general at dermotopes E.11 and U.54. The treatment is bilateral and the action used is anatropic (pricks).

D.39 is then added, always bilaterally, if the pain attacks a lower limb, and E.8 if an upper limb is affected. These dermotopes will be treated twice: first with a catatropic massage which tends to eliminate the accumulated external energy, and then, several days later, after the disappearance (or the alleviation more or less) of the pains, an anatropic action will be used to reinforce the energy system defence mechanism which has failed to repel the invasion due to depletion. Heating is most often employed for this purpose, because pain is a precursor and this signals the presence of *Yang*. If there is no pain, but *Yin*-type signs such as deadness, prick treatment is to be preferred (see Chapter 6).

Specialized Dermotopes
Where symptoms are persistent, a selection should be made from the following specialized dermotopes, according to the region involved:

Shoulder:	E.15, A.12, U.11.
Arm:	E.14.
Elbow:	E.11, R.5.
Forearm:	E.10.
Hip:	B.30.
Thigh:	B.31.
Thigh:	B.31.
Knee	B.34, U.53.
Leg:	U.57, L.6.
Back:	M.13, M.9.
Loins:	U.47, U.25.

Of course, the treatment will be catatropic initially, and afterwards, as the condition improves, the same dermotope will be treated anatropically, for the reasons explained above.

There are no specific dermotopes for the wrists and ankles

and all the local dermotopes can be utilized according to the same method.

In the case of swelling, specific dermotopes are not employed but the dermotopes surrounding the affected region are treated catatropically. Then, but only after the swelling has been resorbed, a start will be made with the treatment described above.

Arthritis deformans is a special case which may be treated without knowing the dermotopes. It is an exception to the rule prohibiting treatment of the *T'ien Ying* points, and it is sufficient to warm the affected joint with the help of a mugwort cigarette (see Chapter 6) until the skin becomes red and *perspires*.

Paresis requires an anatropic action on the dermotopes which control it or the affected muscles, in addition to the usual treatment of the specialized dermotopes. It will be remembered that these *Yin* symptoms call for heat when *Yang* is present (spastic conditions), and for needles if the *Yang* is absent (lax conditions).

Finally, when one is dealing with very muscled regions – the back, in particular – and when the symptoms are not acute and are limited to the superficial layers, a simple cupping-glass is applied to each dermotope of the affected area. In fact, a single cupping-glass is all that is needed, because after being left for a few minutes over one dermotope it can be slid along the skin to the next. The action is a special catatropic one. The displacement of the cupping-glass follows the same rule as that governing the direction of massage.

Dealing with Energy Imbalance

After the patient would have been discharged as cured by Western medicine, the Chinese begin the treatment proper and attack the real cause of the syndrome – the energy imbalance which has made the organism susceptible to adverse atmospheric influences. This imbalance must be corrected if a fairly early relapse is to be avoided.

After equilibration of the peridromes and then of their corresponding functions by way of the cryptodromes, by means of the applications described above, it will be necessary as a logical conclusion of the treatment to deal with certain allodromes (parents of the M. and F. allodromes) which correspond to the neuro-endocrine co-ordinators.

It is astonishing to read in the *Nei Tching Sou Wen* that the sensitivity of the organism to the *Fong Cheu Ping* is primarily caused by 'an insufficiency in the secretion of the *Chen*[1] organ or to an insufficiency in the subtle essence excreted by the brain which stimulates the *Chen* secretion!

If we reword this phrase, which was penned over 4500 years ago, expressing it in up-to-date language, it reads like this: 'The primary cause of the *Fong Cheu Ping* is an insufficiency in the secretion of 11-oxy-steroids by the adrenal cortex (Chen) – that is to say, of hydrocortisone – or else an insufficiency in the secretion of ACTH (this "subtle essence") by the pituitary body (in the brain), the substance which stimulates the adrenal cortex.' One can only be amazed at the clear understanding possessed by the Chinese of the proto-history of these 'subtle essences' which we call hormones and stimulins.

The West shows awareness of these facts when it doses rheumatic subjects with ACTH and corticoids, but fails to appreciate, in spite of its Cartesian logic and rationalism, that the more these substances are supplied to the organism, the more the latter comes to rely on this supplement and the less it will provide the necessary substances for itself. The case is exactly parallel with that of the constipated individual who relies on laxatives. There is a Chinese proverb which says, 'Never give alms, because the recipient will get into the habit of it and will end up by demanding your gift as a right'. A Western doctor remarked to me one day, 'My faith is confined to our marvellous chemical arsenal. Some of my rheumatic

[1] Chen = Kidney

patients have experienced considerable improvement for several years under cortisone.'

In China we call these patients invalids whose improvement is only sustained by what amounts to a glandular prothesis.

What we should be trying to do for preference is to restore a normal secretion of cortisone to the patients. After they think they are cured, we give them two courses of treatment per year for several years in spring and autumn (the seasons when *Yin* and *Yang* are balanced):

Bilateral cauterization of U.23, which, as laboratory controls have shown, stimulates the adrenal secretion, augmenting it as far as 11-oxy-steroids are concerned but not in respect of the other corticosteroids (sexual hormones).

CHAPTER ELEVEN

POINTS OF TECHNIQUE

In micro-massage, treatments are given twice weekly on average, but in certain acute cases the rate of treatment may be increased to as many as two sessions per day.

Although Chinese micro-massage can be considered harmless in general, there are certain precautions which have to be taken in order to avoid the release of energy disturbances which are difficult to reverse.

In the first place it is a general rule that treatment should only be given when the energy is calm. This means that a dermotope must never be touched when energy, whether of the macrocosm or of the microcosm, is being disturbed. The external disturbances (macrocosmic) are wind, rain, thunder, sultry weather, extreme cold and the days of the spring-tide at the seaside. The internal disturbances (microcosmic) are all states of overexcitement, fatigue, grief, vexation, fear, and the menstrual periods. In addition, it is advisable not to treat a pregnant woman or people suffering from cardiovascular trouble in general.

The patient must always be made to lie down at full length.

Also, the prohibitions regarding certain dermotopes as set out in Table 6 should always be borne in mind.

Apart from these precise cases, it must be remembered that it is forbidden to heat dermotopes D.36 and M.22 before the age of seven years at least, it is forbidden to heat F.4 unless the patient has just urinated, and finally it is forbidden to heat F.8 without filling the navel with common salt.

Table 6
Restrictions on anatropic effects

Dermotopes where no heating is allowed: only massage and stimulation with needles are permitted.

R: 3, 8, 10, 11.
E: 19, 20.
D: 7, 8, 9.
L: 1, 7, 9.
A: 9, 18
U: 1, 2, 5, 6, 30, 50, 51, 54, 62.
P: 4, 16, 18, 23.
B: 15, 22, 33, 42.
F: 1.
M: 6, 15, 16, 18, 25.

Dermotopes where no stimulation with needles is allowed: only massage and heating are permitted.

E: 13.
D: 1, 9.
C: 2.
U: 16, 56.
S: 11.
P: 8, 19, 20.
B: 3, 18.
H: 12.
F: 8, 17.
M: 10, 11, 24.

Dermotopes where no heating or stimulation with needles is allowed: only massage is permitted.

D: 17.
M: 7.
M: 17.

Quite aside from the inhibiting effect of certain preliminary treatments,[1] the results obtained by micro-massage are variable, other things being equal, according to the time of treatment. Thus, a cure will require many fewer sessions in spring and autumn than in summer or winter. In spring and autumn, the energy is in a state of balance (50 per cent *Yang* and 50 per cent *Yin*), hence it is easily available. In summer there is too much of it and in winter too little of it. At the

[1] It has now been demonstrated that after treatment with X-rays or even after an ordinary X-ray photo, when corticoids, tranquillizers or hypnotics have been administered, the activity of the dermotopes is very much reduced and often abolished, for a time which varies from several days to several months.

equinoxes (spring and autumn) the energy is like a balance in equilibrium and the least pressure of the thumb, however light, can easily alter this equilibrium; something which calls for a completely different effort at the solstices (summer and winter), when the 'pan of the balance' on which we are acting is either loaded with a maximum weight (summer) or on the contrary with a very light weight (winter).

For the same reason, the most favourable times of day are the morning and the end of the afternoon, which are the hours of energy balance. In addition, it should be remembered that it is unwise to operate on the dermotopes during digestion.

Lastly, and again for the same reasons, the periods of full and new moon are much less favourable than are the periods of the quarters.

Table 7

Time table of the tides of peridromic engery

| Peridrome | Solar hours | |
	Maximum	Minimum
R	4	16
E	6	18
D	8	20
L	10	22
C	12	24
A	14	2
U	16	4
S	18	6
V	20	8
P	22	10
B	24	12
H	2	14

(The allodromes M and F have a constant energy and there is no time-table of quantitative variations for them).

Each peridrome undergoes quantitative variations in energy
in a kind of 'tide' of which the times must be known if one
wishes to profit by these natural movements (Table 7). The
anatropic massage of a given peridrome will have better
results if it is carried out at a 'rising tide' – that is to say,
between the hours of minimum and maximum, whereas
catatropic massage is preferable between the hours of
maximum and minimum at the 'ebb-tide'. For instance,
anatropic massage of a dermotope in the U peridrome is best
done between four and sixteen hours, and its catatropic
massage is best done between sixteen and four hours.

In all cases, after any treatment of a dermotope, the patient
must rest stretched out flat for ten minutes, well covered, and
in a quiet place.

APPENDIX

LOCALIZATION OF THE DERMOTOPES

General Principles Employed in Locating the Dermotopes

The dermotopes, of which the peridromes are the precise alignments, are located by different methods. Apart from anatomical landmarks, intermuscular or intertendinous valleys, or easily palpable depressions such as the subspinous fossa when the arm is raised, the Chinese utilize a system of measures which takes the anatomical 'inch' as its unit (*Ts'oun*). This unit is a relative one with a value which varies from one individual to the other, and even in the same individual according to the region. Figure 9 shows its principal definitions which are:

● The seventh of the distance between the insertion of the deltoid muscle (VD) and the fold of the elbow (PC), measured along the external facies of the arm.
● The twelfth of the distance between the fold of the elbow (PC) and the palmar fold of the wrist (PP), measured along the anterior median line of the forearm.
● The thirteenth of the distance between the prominence of the greater trochanter (GT) and the popliteal fold (fold of the knee, PG), corresponding to the articular interspace, the distance measured along the external facies of the thigh (see supplementary notes later).
● The fifteenth of the distance between the popliteal fold (PG) and the tip of the inner malleolus (ME), measured on

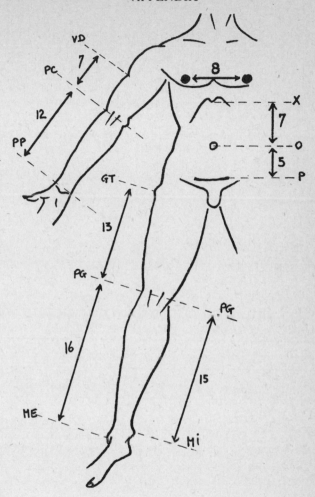

Figure 9
Principal definitions of the Chinese
anatomical 'inch' (Ts'oun)

the internal facies of the leg.

● The sixteenth of the distance between the fold of the knee (PG) and the tip of the outer malleolus (ME), measured on the external facies of the leg.

● The seventh of the distance between the xiphoid appendix (X) and the centre of the navel (O), measured of course along the anterior median line of the trunk.[1]

● The fifth of the distance between the centre of the navel (O) and the superior border of the pubis (P), measured along the median line.

● One forty-second of the waist measurement.

● An eighth of the distance between the two nipples in the man.

Special Rules

In some regions, special rules will help in the measurement of the peridromes. The chief of these rules are the following:

On the thorax, the anterior median line is marked out (allodrome F), then the axillary line, halfway between the anterior and posterior median lines (the latter corresponding to allodrome M).

Halfway between the anterior median and axillary lines is the nipple line (peridrome D).

Halfway between allodrome F (the anterior median line) and peridrome D (the nipple line) is peridrome S.

Halfway between peridrome D (the nipple line) and the axillary line is peridrome L.[2]

In theory, all these alignments are two 'inter-nipple inches' apart. The dermotopes of allodromes S, D and L are situated here in the intercostal spaces and those of allodrome F are on the sternum, on the anterior median line, in the prolongations of the intercostal spaces.

In the back, allodrome M follows the posterior median line,

---

[1] When the xiphoid appendix is absent, count 8 'inches' from the centre of the navel to the inferior border of the sternum.

[2] And, above this, peridrome R begins.

with its interspinous dermotopes.

Parallel to this median posterior line, peridrome U divides into two, between U.11 and U.50, to run in two distinct paths, one external passing inside the internal border of the scapula, the other paramesial, half way between the external path and the median line. Traditionally, there are two 'inches' between the median line and the paramesial path of peridrome U, and two other 'inches' between the latter's paramesial and external paths, when the unit is the 'waist inch'.

The dermotopes of peridrome U are intercostal from U.11 to U.20 and from U.36 to U.44.

On the abdomen, peridromes S, D, L and B are parallel to the median line. Peridrome S runs at a distance of half an 'inch' from this median line; peridrome D runs at a distance of two 'inches' from peridrome S in the extension from the thoracic portion; peridrome L runs at a distance of four 'inches' from peridrome D in the extension from the thoracic portion; and peridrome B (two dermotopes only in this section) runs at a distance of six 'inches' from peridrome L in the extension from the thoracic portion. The unit used here is the 'waist inch'. In a subject of normal build, it is the same as that which defines the distance between the nipples. Some Chinese authors state that all the peridromes are spaced equidistantly on the abdomen at an inch and a half from one another, but this is an approximate measure which should be rejected.

Position of the Dermotopes

All the distal dermotopes, located at the corners of the toe and finger-nails, are found where the two tangents to the midpoints of the bottom and side curves of the nail intersect, as shown in Figure 10.

The paths of the peridromes on the face and cranium have been omitted deliberately here, since they are not used in the practice of massage and kinesitherapy. (However, Figure 11 gives a succinct dermotopic map of the face and head for the sake of completeness.)

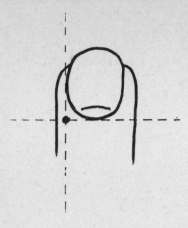

Figure 10
Localization of the distal dermotopes.

Note that the plates at the end of this book are only to be used for micro-massage. *They cannot be employed in acupuncture* BECAUSE THERE IS NO SPECIAL INDICATION OF THOSE DERMOTOPES WHICH MUST NOT BE TREATED BY NEEDLES AND PROBES.

Finally, it will be recalled that all the dermotopes are situated in palpable depressions (*Hsueh*, or 'wells') and that it is absolutely necessary to find them with the finger before starting a treatment because any action outside a dermotope is doomed to failure.

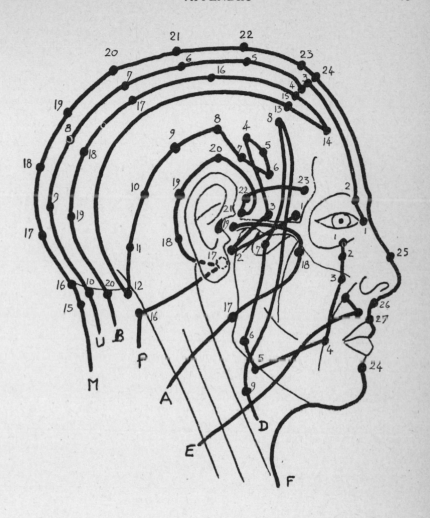

Figure 11
Facial and cranial dermotopes (P.17 is hidden under the ear lobe)

Dermotopes of Peridrome R[3]

Thorax (in line with peridrome L, between the deltoid and the greater pectoral muscles):
R.1: Level with the first intercostal space.
R.2: Under the clavicle.

Anterior facies of the upper arm:
R.3: between the long and the short biceps, one 'inch' below the insertion of the deltoid muscle. (VD).
R.4: between the long and the short biceps, two 'inches' below the insertion of the deltoid muscle (VD).
R.5: in the fold of the elbow, outside the biceps tendon.

Anterior facies of the forearm:
R.6: on the anterior median line of the forearm, between the long supinator and the greater palmar, at seven 'inches' above the level of the palmar fold of the wrist (PP).
R.7: outside the radial artery, two 'inches' above the level of the palmar fold of the wrist (PP).
R.8: Inside the radial artery, one 'inch' above the level of the palmar fold of the wrist (PP).
R.9: Inside the radial artery, in the palmar fold of the wrist (PP).

Palmar facies of the hand:
R.10: Between the first metacarpal and the thenar eminence, halfway between the carpometacarpal and metacarpal-phalangeal joints.
R.11: At the angle of the thumb nail, on the free side (away from the index finger).

Dermotopes of Peridrome E
Dorsal facies of the hand:
E.1: At the angle of the index finger nail, on the thumb side.

[3] See note on page 92 for all points preceded by an asterisk.

E.2: On the external edge of the index finger, where the dorsal skin and the palmar skin meet, in front of the metacarpalphalangeal joint.

E.3: On the external edge, where the dorsal skin and the palmar skin meet, behind the metacarpalphalangeal joint.

E.4: In the angle of the first two metacarpals.

E.5: In the faveola radialis.

External facies of the forearm:

E.6: Three 'inches' above the level of the palmar fold of the wrist (PP), in front of the common extensor, between the long abductor and the short extensor of the thumb.

E.7: Five 'inches' below the level of the fold of the elbow (PC), between the common extensor and the second radial.

E.8: Four 'inches' below the level of the fold of the elbow (PC), between the common extensor and the second radial.

E.9: 'Three 'inches' below the level of the fold of the elbow, between the common extensor and the second radial.

E.10: Two 'inches' below the level of the fold of the elbow, between the common extensor and the second radial.

E.11: At the external extremity of the fold of the elbow in front of the epicondyle, between the first radial and the long supinator.

External facies of the upper arm:

E.12: Two 'inches' above the level of the fold of the elbow (PC), between the long supinator and the anterior brachial muscle.

E.13: Halfway between the level of the fold of the elbow (PC) and the insertion of the deltoid muscle, between the external vastus and the anterior brachial.

E.14: At the point of insertion of the deltoid muscle (VD).

Shoulder and neck:

E.15: Below the acromioclavicular articulation, in a dimple formed when the arm is raised and abducted.

E.16: Inside the acromioclavicular articulation.
*E.17: Between the clavicular and sternal heads of the sternocleidomastoideus muscle, level with the Adam's apple.
*E.18: Between the clavicular and sternal heads of the sternum, at the level of the hyoid bone.

(From there the peridrome E passes to the face, where it has two dermotopes).

Dermotopes of Peridrome D

(This peridrome starts in the face, where it has eight dermotopes).

Neck:
D.9: On the carotid pulse, in front of the sternocleido-mastoideus muscle.
D.10: Between the sternocleidomastoideus muscle and the thyroid cartilage, at the level of the Adam's apple.
D.11: Above the clavicle, between the sternal and clavicular heads of the sternocleidomastoideus muscle.
D.12: Above the clavicle between the trapezius and the clavicular head of the sternocleidomastoideus muscle.

Thorax (line running down through nipple)
D.13: Between the clavicle and the first rib.
D.14: In the first intercostal space.
D.15: In the second intercostal space.
D.16: In the third intercostal space.
D.17: In the fourth intercostal space (nipple).
D.18: In the fifth intercostal space.

Abdomen (two 'inches' away from the anterior median line)
D.19: Six 'inches' above the O (navel) level.
D.20: Five 'inches' above the O level.
D.21: Four 'inches' above the O level.
D.22: Three 'inches' above the O level.
D.23: Two 'inches' above the O level.

D.24: One 'inch' above the O level.

D.25: Level with the navel.

D.26: One 'inch' below the O level.

D.27: Two 'inches' below the O level.

D.28: Three 'inches' below the O level.

D.29: Four 'inches' below the O level.

D.30: Five 'inches' below the O level above the superior border of the pubic bone.

Anteroexternal facies of the thigh:

*D.31: level with the greater trochanter (GT), outside the anterior rectus.

*D.32: Seven 'inches' above the fold of the Knee (PG), outside the anterior rectus.

*D.33: Five 'inches' above the level of the fold of the Knee (PG) outside the anterior rectus.

*D.34: Four 'inches' above the level of the fold of the Knee (PG) outside the anterior rectus.

D.35: Outside the patellar tendon, level with the intercondylar line.

Anteroexternal facies of the leg:

D.36: Between the tibia and the anterior tibial muscle, three 'inches' below the fold of the knee. (PG).

D.37: Between the tibia and the anterior tibial muscle, six 'inches' below the fold of the knee. (PG).

D.38: Between the tibia and the anterior tibial muscle, eight 'inches' below the fold of the knee (PG).

D.39: Between the tibia and the anterior tibial muscle, nine 'inches' below the fold of the knee.

*D.40: Between the anterior tibial muscle and the common extensor, level with D.39.

Dorsal facies of the foot:

D.41: In the centre of the instep, level with the MI, between the tendons of the common extensor and the special extensor of the great toe.

D.42: In the metatarsal, on the articulation between calcaneum, cuboid, talus, and scaphoid.

D.43: In the angle of the second and third metatarsals.

D.44: Interdigital space between the second and third toes.

D.45: At the angle of the second toe-nail, next to the third toe.

Internal facies of the foot:

L.1: At the angle of the big toe-nail on the inner side of the foot.

L.2: At the border between the dorsal and plantar skin, in front of the metatarsophalangeal joint of the first toe.

L.3: At the border between the dorsal and plantar skin, behind the metatarsophalangeal joint of the first toe.

L.4: At the border between the dorsal and plantar skin, under the centre of the first metatarsal.

L.5: In front of and below the MI, on the line of the articulation between the talus and the scaphoid.

Internal facies of the leg:

*L.6: Behind the tibia, four 'inches' above the level of the MI.

*L.7: Behind the tibia, seven 'inches' above the level of the MI.

*L.8: Behind the tibia, nine 'inches' above the level of the MI.

*L.9: On the tibia, under 'crow's feet'.

Anterointernal facies of the thigh:

*L.10: Between the sartorius and the internal rectus, four 'inches' above the level of the fold of the knee.

*L.11: In the inferior angle of Scarpa's triangle, eight 'inches' above the level of the fold of the knee.

L.12: In the fold of the groin, four 'inches' from the median line (pubic level).

Abdomen (four 'inches' from the median line):

L.13: One 'inch' above the pubic level (P).

L.14: One 'inch' below the level of the navel (O).

L.15: Level with the navel.

L.16: Three 'inches' above the level of the navel. According to the form of the costal border, this dermotope can be either abdominal or thoracic.

Thorax (halfway between peridrome D and the axillary line):

L.17: In the fifth intercostal space.

L.18: In the fourth intercostal space.

L.19: In the third intercostal space.

L.20: In the second intercostal space.

Axillary line:

L.21: On the axillary line, in the tenth intercostal space.

Dermotopes of Peridrome C

Axillary fossa:

C.1: At the bottom of the axillary fossa.

Anterointernal facies of the upper arm:

C.2: Between the biceps and the anterior brachial, three 'inches' above the level of the fold of the elbow.

C.3: Towards the internal extremity of the fold of the elbow, in front of the epitrochlea, on the insertion of the round pronator.

Anterior facies of the forearm:

C.4: In the cubital fossa, one 'inch' and a half above the palmar fold of the wrist (PP).

C.5: In the cubital fossa, one 'inch' above the palmar fold of the wrist (PP).

C.6: In the cubital fossa, half an 'inch' above the palmar fold of the wrist (PP).

C.7: In the cubital fossa, in the fold of the wrist.

Palmar facies of the hand:
C.8: In the palm, between the fourth and fifth metacarpals, on the upper transverse line.

Dorsal facies of the hand:
C.8: At the angle of the little finger nail next to the ring finger.

Dermotopes of Peridrome A

Cubital border of the hand:
A.1: At the angle of the little finger nail on the cubital side.
A.2: On the border between the palmar and dorsal skin, in front of the metacarpophalangeal joint of the little finger.
A.3: On the border between the palmar and dorsal skin, behind the metacarpophalangeal joint of the little finger.
A.4: On the border between the palmar and dorsal skin, under the pisiform bone.
*A.5: In the dorsal fold of the wrist, under the cubital styloid.

Posterior facies of the forearm:
A.6: Two 'inches' above the level of the fold or the wrist (PP), between the tendon of the common extensor and the radial border of the cubitus.
A.7: Five 'inches' above the level of the fold of the wrist (PP), and inside the cubitus.

Posterior facies of the upper arm:
A.8: At the level of the fold of the elbow (PP), inside the olecranon, on the cubital.
*A.9: One 'inch' above the insertion of the deltoid muscle (VD), under the border of the deltoid, between the vastus externus and the long portion of the triceps.

Posterior facies of the shoulder:
A.10: Under the acromion, on the glenohumeral articulation.
A.11: In the centre of the subspinous fossa.[4]

A.12: In the coracoid notch.[4]
A.13: In the centre of the supra-spinous fossa.[4]
A.14: Above U.36, level with U.11.
A.15: On a vertical passing half way between the two pathways of peridrome U, level with the spinal equivalent of C.7.

Neck:
*A.16: Behind the sternocleidomastoideus muscle, level with E.18.
(From here, peridrome A goes to the face, where it has three dermotopes).

Dermotopes of Peridrome U
(This peridrome starts at the face, then passes to the cranium, and has nine dermotopes in these areas).

Neck (*rear facies*):
U.10: Under the occipital base, halfway between M.16 and B.20.

Paramesial dorsal course:
U.11: Level with the interspinal space D1-D2.
U.12: Level with the interspinal space D2-D3.
U.13: Level with the interspinal space D3-D4.
U.14: Level with the interspinal space D4-D5.
U.15: Level with the interspinal space D5-D6.
U.16: Level with the interspinal space D6-D7.
U.17: Level with the interspinal space D7-D8.
U.18: Level with the interspinal space D9-D10.
U.19: Level with the interspinal space D10-D11.
U.20: Level with the interspinal space D11-D12.
U.21: Level with the interspinal space D12-L1.
U.22: Level with the interspinal space L1-L2.

[4] In a dimple formed when the arm is raised.

U.23: Level with the interspinal space L2-L3.
U.24: Level with the interspinal space L3-L4.
U.25: Level with the interspinal space L4-L5.
U.26: Above the sacro-iliac articulation.
U.27: Under the sacro-iliac, level with the first sacral foramen.[5]
U.28: On the border of the sacrum, level with the second sacral foramen.[5]
U.29: On the border of the sacrum, level with the third sacral foramen.[5]
U.30: On the border of the sacrum, level with the fourth sacral foramen.[5]
U.31: In the first sacral foramen.
U.32: In the second sacral foramen.
U.33: In the third sacral foramen.
U.34: In the fourth sacral foramen.
U.35: Outside the sacrococcygeal articulation.

External dorsal course:
U.36: Level with U.12.
U.37: Level with U.13.
U.38: Level with U.14.
U.39: Level with U.15.
U.40: Level with U.16.
U.41: Level with U.17.
U.42: Level with U.18.
U.43: Level with U.19.
U.44: Level with U.20.
U.45: Level with U.21.
U.46: Level with U.22.
U.47: Level with U.23.
U.48: Level with U.28.
U.49: Level with U.30.

[5] (1) Always two 'inches' from the posterior median line.

Posterior facies of the thigh:

U.50: Between the cnemial biceps and the semitendinous muscle, in the fold of the buttocks, about three 'inches' below the level of the greater trochanter (GT).

*U.51: Between the cnemial biceps and the semitendinous muscle, six 'inches' below the level of the greater trochanter (GT).

U.52: Inside the tendon of the cnemial biceps, one 'inch' above the level of the greater trochanter (GT).

U.53: Inside the tendon of the cnemial biceps, in the popliteal fold.

U.54: In the centre of the popliteal fold

Posterior facies of the lower leg:

U.55: Between the gemellus muscles, two 'inches' below the fold of the knee (PG).

U.56: Between the gemellus muscles, four 'inches' below the fold of the knee (PG).

U.57: Between the gemellus muscles, seven 'inches' below the level of the fold of the knee (PG).

External facies of the lower leg:

U.58: In front of the Achilles tendon, eight 'inches' above the external malleolus (ME) (seven 'inches' according to some Chinese authors).

U.59: In front of the Achilles tendon, three 'inches' above the level of the external malleolus (ME).

External facies of the foot:

U.60: Behind and on a level with the external malleolus.

U.61: In the middle of the calcaneum.

U.62: Under the external malleolus.

U.63: In front of and below the external malleolus.

U.64: On the border between the dorsal and plantar skin, behind the tubercle of the fifth metatarsal.

U.65: On the border of the dorsal and plantar skin, behind the metatarsophalangeal articulation of the fifth toe.

U.66: On the border between the dorsal and plantar skin, in front of the metatarsophalangeal articulation of the fifth toe.
U.67: At the angle of the fifth toe-nail, on the other side.

Plantar facies of the foot:
S.1: In the centre of the ball of the foot.
S.2: Under the articulation between the scaphoid and the first cuneiform bone.
S.3: Behind and level with the internal malleolus.
S.4: On the superior border of the calcaneum.
S.5: In the centre of the calcaneum.
S.6: Under the internal malleolus.

Internal facies of the lower leg:
*S.7: In front of the Achilles tendon, three 'inches' above the level of the internal malleolus (MI).
*S.8: Behind the tibia, three 'inches' above the level of the internal malleolus (MI).
*S.9: In front of the Achilles tendon, six 'inches' above the level of the internal malleolus (MI).
S.10: Level with the popliteal fold between the semitendinous muscle and the internal rectus.
(Peridrome S has no dermotopes on the thigh).

Abdomen (half an 'inch' from the median line):
S.11: On the superior border of the pubis.
S.12: One 'inch' above the pubis.
S.13: Two 'inches' above the pubis.
S.14: Three 'inches' above the pubis.
S.15: Four 'inches' above the pubis.
S.16: Level with the navel.
S.17: Two 'inches' above the navel level.
S.18: Three 'inches' above the navel level.
S.19: Four 'inches' above the navel level.
S.20: Five 'inches' above the navel level.
S.21: Six 'inches' above the navel level.

Thorax (halfway between the median line and the vertical line running through the nipple):
S.22: In the fifth intercostal space.
S.23: In the fourth intercostal space.
S.24: In the third intercostal space.
S.25: In the second intercostal space.
S.26: In the first intercostal space.
S.27: Between the clavicle and the first rib.

Dermotopes of Peridrome V
Thorax:
V.1: In the fourth intercostal space, halfway between D 17 and L.18.

Anterior facies of the arm:
V.2: Level with the insertion of the deltoid muscle (VD), between the biceps and the anterior brachial muscle.
V.3: In the fold of the elbow, inside the tendon of the biceps.

Anterior facies of the forearm.
V.4: Below R.6, between the longer and shorter palmar muscles, five 'inches' above the level of the fold of the wrist (PP).
V.5: Below R.6, between the longer and shorter palmar muscles, three 'inches' above the level of the fold of the wrist (PP).
V.6: Below R.6, between the longer and shorter palmar muscles, two 'inches' above the level of the fold of the wrist (PP).
V.7: In the centre of the fold of the wrist.

Palmar facies of the hand:
V.8: In the centre of the palm, between the third and fourth metacarpals, on the lower transverse line.
V.9: In the angle of the middle finger-nail, next to the index finger.

Dermotopes of Peridrome P

Dorsal facies of the hand

P.1: In the angle of the ring finger-nail, next to the little finger.

P.2: In the interdigital space between the ring and the little fingers.

P.3: Between the fourth and fifth metacarpals, behind the metacarpophalangeal articulations.

P.4: In the centre of the dorsal fold of the wrist.

Posterior facies of the forearm:

P.5: On the posterior median line of the forearm, two 'inches' above the level of the fold of the wrist (PP).

P.6: Inside the cubital border of the radius, three 'inches' above the level of the fold of the wrist (PP).

P.7: Outside the radial border of the cubitus, three 'inches' above the level of the fold of the wrist (PP).

P.8: Between the radius and the cubitus, four 'inches' above the level of the fold of the wrist (PP).

P.9: Between the radius and the cubitus, six 'inches' above the level of the fold of the wrist (PP).

Posterior facies of the arm:

P.10: One-and-a-half 'inches' approximately above the level of the fold of the elbow (PC), outside the tendon of the triceps, above the trochlea.[6]

P.11: Two-and-a-half 'inches' approximately above the level of the fold of the elbow (PC), outside the tendon of the triceps.[6]

P.12: At the insertion of the external vastus and of the long triceps in their common tendon, two 'inches' below the level of the insertion of the deltoid muscle.

---

[6] According to some Chinese authors, P.10 and P.11 are inside the tendon, and this seems to be more accurate.

Posterior facies of the shoulder:
*P.13: On the humerus, between the external vastus and the long triceps (which can be perceived in relief even though it passes under the deltoid muscle), level with A.11.
P.14: Under the acromion, outside the humerus.
P.15: Vertically above A.13, level with the 'spinal' C.7. (From here, peridrome P passes to the face, where it has eight dermotopes).

Dermotopes of Peridrome B
(This peridrome starts in the face and then passes to the cranium along a complex route, covering nineteen dermotopes in its course).

Neck and shoulder:
B.20: Under the occipital base, between the trapezius and the sternocleidomastoideus muscle.
B.21: At the base of the neck, in front of the trapezius, on the intermediate cervical sympathic ganglion.

Thorax:
B.22: On the axillary line, in the fourth intercostal space.
B.23: In the fourth intercostal space, halfway between B.22 and L.18.
B.24: In the seventh intercostal space on the line running down through the nipple.

Abdomen:
B.25: In front of the tip of the twelfth rib.
B.26: On the axillary line, above the iliac crest.
B.27: Six 'inches' from the anterior median line and two 'inches' above the pubic level (P).
B.28: Six 'inches' from the median anterior line and one 'inch' above the pubic level (P).

External facies of the thigh:

B.29: In front of and level with the greater trochanter.

B.30: Behind and about an 'inch' below the prominence of the greater trochanter.

*B.31: Between the ischiatic portion of the cnemial biceps and the external vastus, six 'inches' above the level of the fold of the knee.

*B.32: Between the ischiatic portion of the cnemial biceps and the external vastus, five 'inches' above the level of the fold of the knee (PG).

*B.33: One 'inch' above the level of the fold of the knee (PG) and above the external condyle.

External facies of the lower leg:

*B.34: Three 'inches' below the fold of the knee (PG), on the head of the fibula, between the long peroneal and the soleus muscles.

B.35: Seven 'inches' above the external malleolus (ME), between the long peroneal and soleus muscles.

B.36: Seven 'inches' above the external malleolus (ME), between the long peroneal and the common extensor.

B.37: Five 'inches' above the level of the external malleolus, between the long peroneal and the common extensor.

B.38: Four 'inches' above the level of the external malleolus, between the common extensor and the anterior tibial muscle.

B.39: Three 'inches' above the level of the external malleolus, between the long peroneal and the common extensor.

Dorsal facies of the foot:

B.40: In front of and level with the external malleolus.

B.41: In the angle of the fourth and fifth metatarsals.

B.42: Between the fourth and fifth metatarsals, behind the metatarsophalangeal articulations.

B.43: In the interdigital space between the fourth and fifth toes.

B.44: In the angle of the fourth toe-nail next the fifth toe.

Dermotopes of Peridrome H

Dorsal facies of the foot:
H.1: In the angle of the nail of the big toe, next to the second toe.
H.2: In the interdigital space between the first two toes.
H.3: In the angle between the first two metatarsals.
H.4: Halfway between the internal malleolus and D.41.

Internal facies of the lower leg:
*H.5: Behind the tibia, six 'inches' above the level of the internal malleolus (MI).
*H.6: Behind the tibia, eight 'inches' above the level of the internal malleolus (MI).
H.7: Behind the tibia, three 'inches' below the level of the fold of the knee (PG).
H.8: Level with the fold of the knee between the internal rectus and the sartorius.

Anterointernal facies of the thigh:
*H.9: Behind the sartorius muscle, five 'inches' above the fold of the knee (PG).
H.10: On the femoral pulse, one 'inch' above the greater trochanter (GT).
H.11: On the femoral pulse, level with the greater trochanter (GT), in the fold of the groin.
H.12: In the fold of the groin, halfway between H.12 and L.12.

Abdomen:
H.13: In front of the tip of the eleventh rib.

Thorax:
H.14: On the vertical line through the nipple in the sixth intercostal space.

Dermotopes of Allodrome F

Perineum:
F.1: In the centre of the perineum.

Abdomen (median line):
F.2: Just above the upper border of the pubis.
F.3: One 'inch' above the pubic level (P).
F.4: Two 'inches' above the pubic level (P).
F.5: Three 'inches' above the pubic level (P).
F.6: Three-and-a-half 'inches' above the pubic level (P).
F.7: Four 'inches' above the pubic level (P).
F.8: The centre of the navel.
F.9: Pne 'inch' above the navel (O).
F.10: Two 'inches' above the navel (O).
F.11: Three 'inches' above the navel (O).
F.12: Four 'inches' above the navel (O).
F.13: Five 'inches' above the navel (O).
F.14: Six 'inches' above the navel (O).
F.15: Below the extremity of the xiphoid appendix, or one 'inch' below the inferior border of the sternum, if this appendix is missing.

Thorax (anterior median line):
F.16: In the prolongation of the fifth intercostal space.
F.17: In the prolongation of the fourth intercostal space.
F.18: In the prolongation of the third intercostal space.
F.19: In the prolongation of the second intercostal space.
F.20: In the prolongation of the first intercostal space.
F.21: In the prolongation of the space between the clavicle and the first rib.

Neck:
F.22: Just above the sternal notch.
F.23: On the hyoid bone.
(From here, the allodrome F goes to the face, where it has its final dermotope).

Dermotopes of Allodrome M
Lumbosacral region (median line):
M.1: Under the tip of the coccyx.
M.2: On the sacrococcygeal articulation.
M.3: In the interspinous space L4-L5.
M.4: In the interspinous space L2-L3.
M.5: In the interspinous space L1-L2.

Dorsal region (median line):
M.6: In the interspinous space D11-D12.
M.7: In the interspinous space D10-D11.
M.8: In the interspinous space D9-D10.
M.9: In the interspinous space D7-D8.
M.10: In the interspinous space D6-D7.
M.11: In the interspinous space D5-D6.
M.12: In the interspinous space D3-D4.
M.13: In the interspinous space D1-D2.

Neck: (posterior median line):
M.14: In the interspinous space C7-D1.
M.15: Level with the atlas.
M.16: Under the occipital base.
(From here, allodrome M passes to the cranium and the face,
where it has its twelve last dermotopes).

SUPPLEMENTARY NOTES

According to the classical texts of Chinese acupuncture, the length of the thigh is thirteen 'inches' compared with that of the lower leg. The fact of the matter is that in the occidental races, and also in the inhabitants of Northern China (who are of mixed Chinese, Turkish and Mongolian descent), the femur is longer, other things being equal, than in the pure Chinese of the South or in the Japanese. Hence it is now accepted that in races with 'a long femur', the measure is fifteen 'inches' between the greater trochanter (GT) and the fold of the knee (PG).

It is also worth mentioning that on the occasion of my last visit to China in 1967, we had the opportunity of examining certain proposed dermotope localizations which are still being debated in various schools. Without attempting to take sides, I shall give here the corrections advocated by certain Chinese authorities.

These alternative dermotope localizations are the following: E.17 and E.18 are said to be behind the sternocleido-mastoideus muscle.

D.31 is placed an 'inch' lower down, i.e. one 'inch' below the level of the greater trochanter (GT).

D.32 is nine 'inches' below the level of the greater trochanter (GT), i.e. six 'inches' above the fold of the knee (PG).

D.33 is three 'inches' above the level of the fold of the knee (PG), i.e. twelve 'inches' below the level of the greater trochanter (GT).

D.34 is two 'inches' above the fold of the knee (PG), i.e. thirteen 'inches' below the level of the greater trochanter

(GT).

D.40 is level with D.38, eight 'inches' from the external malleolus (ME) and from the fold of the knee (PG).

L.6 is three 'inches' from the internal malleolus (MI).

L.7 is six 'inches' from the internal malleolus (MI).

L.8 is ten 'inches' from the internal malleolus (MI).

L.9 is one 'inch' under the fold of the knee (inter-line).

L.10 is two 'inches' above the level of the fold of the knee.

L.11 is ten 'inches' above the fold of the knee, i.e. five 'inches' below the greater trochanter (GT).

A.5 is on the cubital facies of the wrist, on the inter-cubitocarpal line, symmetrical with the faveola radialis – E.5.

A.9 is located towards the extremity of the axillary fold, between the external border of the scapula and the border of the deltoid.

A.16 would be in front of the trapezius, behind E.18, which is behind the sternocleidomastoideus muscle.

U.51 is nine 'inches' under the greater trochanter (GT), i.e. six 'inches' above the level of the fold of the knee (PG).

S.7 is two 'inches' above the internal malleolus (MI).

S.8 is two 'inches' above the internal malleolus (MI).

S.9 is six 'inches' above the internal malleolus (MI).

P.13 although still found between the two muscles, is under the deltoid (where A.9 is on the plate).

B.31 is six 'inches' from the fold of the knee (PG), i.e. nine 'inches' from the greater trochanter (GT).

B.32 is five 'inches' from the fold of the knee (PG), i.e. ten 'inches' from the greater trochanter (GT).

B.33 is two 'inches' from the fold of the knee (PG), thirteen 'inches' from the greater trochanter (GT).

B.34 would be one 'inch' under the fold of the knee (PG) (inter-line), above the head of the fibula.

H.5 is five 'inches' from the internal malleolus (MI).

H.6 is seven 'inches' from the internal malleolus (MI).

H.9 is four 'inches' from the fold of the knee (PG), i.e. eleven 'inches' from the greater trochanter (GT).

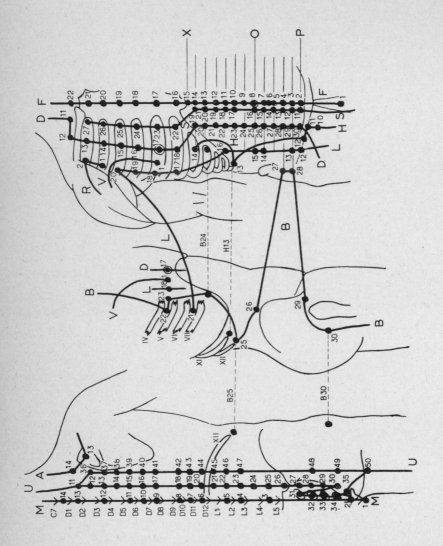

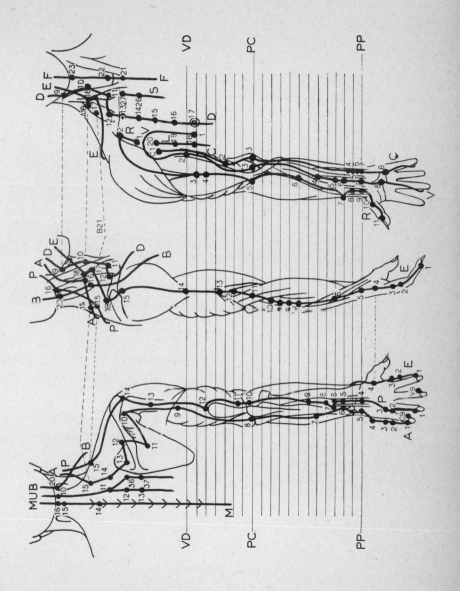

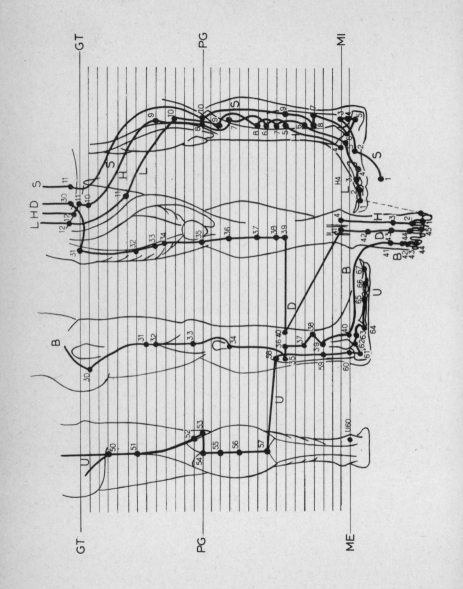